Episiotomy

Challenging Obstetric Interventions

Episiotomy
Challenging Obstetric Interventions

Ian D. Graham
PhD, MA, BA

Clinical Epidemiology Unit
Ottawa Civic Hospital Loeb Research Institute

Blackwell
Science

© 1997 by
Blackwell Science Ltd
Editorial Offices:
Osney Mead, Oxford OX2 0EL
25 John Street, London WC1N 2BL
23 Ainslie Place, Edinburgh EH3 6AJ
350 Main Street, Malden
   MA 02148 5018, USA
54 University Street, Carlton
   Victoria 3053, Australia

Other Editorial Offices:

Blackwell Wissenschafts-Verlag GmbH
   Kurfürstendamm 57
   10707 Berlin, Germany

Zehetnergasse 6
A-1140 Wien
Austria

First published 1997

Set in 10 on 11½ Palatino
by DP Photosetting, Aylesbury, Bucks
Printed and bound in Great Britain by
Hartnolls Ltd, Bodmin, Cornwall

The Blackwell Science logo is a
trade mark of Blackwell Science Ltd,
registered at the United Kingdom
Trade Marks Registry

DISTRIBUTORS
Marston Book Services Ltd
PO Box 269
Abingdon
Oxon OX14 4YN
(*Orders:* Tel: 01235 465500
          Fax: 01235 465555)

USA
Blackwell Science, Inc.
Commerce Place
350 Main Street
Malden, MA 02148 5018
(*Orders:* Tel: 800 759 6102
          617 388 8250
     Fax: 617 388 8255)

Canada
Copp Clark Professional
200 Adelaide Street, West, 3rd Floor
Toronto, Ontario M5H 1W7
(*Orders:* Tel: 416 597-1616
          800 815-9417
     Fax: 416 597-1617)

Australia
Blackwell Science Pty Ltd
54 University Street
Carlton, Victoria 3053
(*Orders:* Tel: 03 9347 0300
     Fax: 03 9347 5001)

A catalogue record for this title
is available from the British Library

ISBN 0-632-04145-5

Library of Congress
Cataloging-in-Publication Data
Graham, Ian D.
   Episiotomy: challenging obstetric
interventions/Ian D. Graham.
      p. cm.
   Originally presented as the author's
thesis (Ph.D.).
   Includes bibliographical references
and index.
   ISBN 0-632-04145-5
   1. Episiotomy—History. I. Title.
   {DNLM: 1. Episiotomy—history—
United States. 2. Episiotomy—history
—Great Britain.   WQ 11 AA1
G7e 1997]
RG791.G73 1997
618.8'5—dc20
DNLM/DLC
for Library of Congress   96-43827
                                         CIP

For Dawn
and
Jordi

Contents

Contents

Foreword

Murray W. Enkin, MD, FRCS(c), Professor Emeritus,
Departments of Obstetrics & Gynaecology, Clinical Epidemiology
and Biostatistics, McMaster University, Canada

Episiotomy: Challenging Obstetric Interventions is a remarkably well-researched and well-written history of 'the unkindest cut of all'. It provides valuable insights into the pace and process of change and the factors that promote and inhibit it.

Current models of medicine encompass two archetypes: medicine as science and medicine as art. We combine in our imagination pictures of the white-coated doctor in the laboratory and the kindly family physician at the bedside. These models reassure and comfort us. They tell us that our doctors will use their science to practise the most effective care available and their art to meet our needs as individuals.

Both these models are useful, and at least partially valid. The role of science in medicine cannot be disputed. Basic and directed scientific research has produced important medical advances. Controlled studies have provided unbiased evidence about the effects of many medical practices and procedures, and this evidence is disseminated throughout the world through the efforts of the international Cochrane Collaboration. Nor can the art of medicine be ignored. Effective care cannot be reduced to simple algorithms. Doctors do care, and realize that the important thing is to treat the patient rather than the disease.

These archetypes also have some serious flaws. Medicine is not a science, because science is inherently reproducible and universal. Scientific evidence cannot be ignored; the laws of physics are recognized and accepted by scientists from Australia to Zimbabwe. Similarly human physiology is the same the world over, and the same medical literature, with the same evidence, is available to all; yet treatments for the same condition vary from country to country, from institution to institution, from doctor to doctor. These variations in clinical policy are far too great to explain by differences in the populations served or the resources available, and they challenge the image of medicine as a science. Nor can we fall back on the view of medicine as an art as a satisfactory explanation of these variations in practice. Often what is labelled as the art of medicine is merely an unthinking implementation of lessons learned from teachers in medical school, from the unsubstantiated opinions of 'expert' authorities, or from fallible personal experience.

The incomplete nature of both the science and art models of medicine suggest that we look for a different metaphor, one which more closely accords with what we actually observe. Perhaps a more accurate (although less comforting) complementary model might be to consider medicine as a 'fashion' (or one of its synonyms, such as 'custom', 'fad', 'mode', 'vogue'). The fashion model would recognize that technologies can be introduced, become accepted as fashionable, then conventional, then be rejected, and decline or disappear, with little or no scientific justification.

The model of medicine as fashion serves a useful descriptive function, and shows us that we have to look beyond science or art to explain the geographic and secular shifting trends in medical policies. But even this does not explain exactly how or why some practices rise and flourish, while others wither early on the vine. Those who would like to see medical practice truly become a science and an art must first try to understand the complex causal web of clinical policy. Why do we do what we do?

There is little direct evidence of how or why changes in medical practice occur. Evidence published in the medical literature is ignored, often for decades. Clinical guidelines proposed by experts and promulgated by official or national bodies have had little discernible effect on practice, although they may predispose to later change. Local initiatives, using local opinion leaders, can have a major effect in a particular setting, but little effect on the wider community. In the absence of experimental evidence about how to bring about change we must rely on observation, on careful analysis of the history and sociology of medical innovation. By learning about the forces that have influenced the initiation and utilization of particular interventions in the past, we may gain insights and be able to formulate general rules which can be applied to other situations in the present and future.

In this book, Ian Graham has carried out a socio-historical analysis of the rise and fall of a particular low-tech obstetrical intervention. Episiotomy, the operation he has chosen for study, was introduced to be occasionally used in emergency situations, but came to be used almost universally. The procedure, while simple, is far from innocuous. It causes discomfort to many women, and serious sequelae to some. It came into widespread use without scientifically based evidence of benefit. Who were its proponents, who were its publicizers? Why were they so successful? How?

Perhaps even more importantly, the practice of episiotomy came under closer scrutiny, began to be questioned, and in some countries its use rapidly declined. What sparked that scrutiny? Who initiated the questioning? And how did the profession respond? This book provides answers to these questions.

Episiotomy is important in itself, as a significant factor affecting women's comfort and health after childbirth. It is important also as a symbol, as an example of a medical fashion that arose, burgeoned, proliferated, and flourished without recourse to either science or art; and which was successfully challenged by those who used both art and science to change the direction of the juggernaut.

We have much to learn from this meticulously researched story. It is a great piece of work, and essential reading for all those involved in effecting change within midwifery and obstetrical practice and management.

Acknowledgements

As with any undertaking of this type, there have been dozens, perhaps hundreds, of individuals who have helped me with my research in one way or another over the past several years. They have furnished data, conducted searches of the literature, located and retrieved ancient texts, translated documents, prepared figures and tables, offered valuable insights, challenged my interpretations, read and commented on drafts of chapters, provided encouragement, and supported me financially and emotionally. To all of these individuals I owe a great deal. Without them this book would not be as it is.

I am particularly indebted to Beverley Lawrence Beech, Dean Fergusson, Sara Frisch, Sheila Kitzinger, Andreas Laupacis, Jo Logan, Flo Tracy, Wikke Walop, Vivienne Walters and Karen Weeks. The last chapter of the book is co-authored by Barbara Davies, PhD (candidate), MScN, BScN, RN, an Assistant Professor in the School of Nursing at the University of Ottawa; I am grateful to Barbara for taking time away from her doctoral research to collaborate with me in writing this chapter. I also owe an enormous intellectual debt to my doctoral thesis supervisor, Jim Robbins, and my other committee members, Joan Stelling and Prue Rains, for encouraging me to question everything that is taken for granted. Joan and Jim's careful editing has made this work much more logical and readable.

Another group of individuals who deserve special recognition are my key informants. These individuals gave more generously of their time than I could have ever hoped for. In addition to sitting for the interview, many also helped arrange interviews with others, opened their files to me, or sent me documents and information they thought would be useful.

I am also very grateful to Lisa Field and Griselda Campbell, Publishers at Blackwell Science, for believing that my thesis should be turned into a book and to Sarah-Kate Powell, Development Editor at Blackwell Science, for seeing that this happened in a very timely manner. I would also like to thank the individuals who reviewed the work for Blackwell Science for their helpful advice and suggestions.

Had it not been for a number of generous benefactors, this research would not have come to fruition. I have been supported in part by funding from a J.W. McConnell Memorial Fellowship, a Birks Family Foundation Fellowship, a McGill University Humanities and Social Science Research Grant, a Government of Quebec FCAR PhD Fellowship, a National Health Research and Development Programme of Canada PhD Fellowship, and a Medical Research Council of Canada Post Doctoral Health Research Fellowship. The Clinical Epidemiology Unit of the Loeb Research Institute of the Ottawa Civic Hospital has also been very supportive of this endeavour.

Finally, I owe so much to my family. My parents, Fern and Doug, my wife's parents, Murielle and George, and Dawn and Tony whom we have come to think of as our adoptive English parents, have encouraged and supported this effort in many different ways over the years. Our son Jordi has been very forgiving of his father spending so much time working on this book. As for Dawn, my wife, her patience and encouragement have been exceptional and unfaltering and her research assistance truly invaluable. Without her, this work would probably not have been undertaken or completed.

List of Abbreviations

AAOG	American Association of Obstetricians and Gynecologists
ABOG	American Board of Obstetrics and Gynecology
AGS	American Gynecological Society
AIMS	Association for Improvements in the Maternity Services
ARM	artificial rupture of the membranes
ASPO	American Society for Psychoprophylaxis in Obstetrics
BMJ	British Medical Journal
CAS	Current Awareness Service
CQA	continuous quality assurance
CQI	continuous quality improvement
DHSS	Department of Health and Social Services
DES	diethylstilbestrol
ECPC	Effective care in pregnancy and childbirth
GECPC	Guide to effective care in pregnancy and childbirth
HES	Hospital Episode System
HIPE	Maternity Hospital In-patient Enquiry
ICEA	International Childbirth Education Association
MDF	Maternity Defence Fund
MIDIRS	Midwives Information and Resources Service
MIRIAD	Midwifery Research Database
NAPCRG	North American Primary Care Research Group
NAPSAC	National Association of Parents and Professionals for Safe Alternatives in Childbirth
NCT	National Childbirth Trust
NPEU	National Perinatal Epidemiology Unit
OTA	Office of Technology Assessment
RCTs	randomized controlled trials

Introduction

'These pages have not been written for those who lay them aside saying or thinking, "Much ado about a perineal tear!" They will have to come to terms with their own consciences.' (Ritgen, 1855 (translated by Wynn, 1965:433))

How and why does obstetrical orthodoxy and use of obstetric interventions change over time? How do obstetric interventions come into vogue and become standard or routine practice? Why do they lose favour and eventually get abandoned? What role does scientific evidence play in bringing about these changes? How long does it take? What non-medical and non-scientific factors are implicated in the process and how important are they in bringing about change in obstetric interventions?

This book sets out to answer these questions by studying the process of change in one particular obstetrical intervention: episiotomy. Episiotomy, or more appropriately perineotomy, is the surgical enlargement of the birth canal made at the time of birth, presumably to facilitate the birth. The operation is performed with a pair of scissors or a scalpel. The two most common types of episiotomy are midline or median and mediolateral (Fig. 1). Midline or median episiotomies are favoured in the USA and Canada while mediolateral ones are more commonly performed in the UK.

Inevitably, one of the first questions I am asked when I present my research is why a male sociologist would be interested in episiotomy. The answer is that I was fortunate enough to be in the right place at the right time. While working on course work for my doctorate at McGill University in Montreal, I became interested in the process by which medical technology is developed and changed. Around 1987 when I was looking for a dissertation topic, physicians at McGill University and the Université de Montréal collaborated on a randomized controlled trial of episiotomy. I became aware of this trial when one of my professors, who later became my thesis supervisor, gave me the study grant proposal to read. As I read through the proposal I was struck that what was being proposed was a study to evaluate an obstetrical pro-

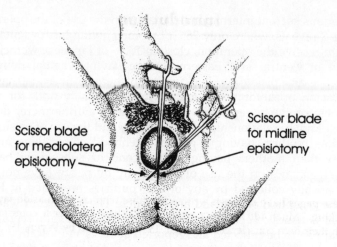

Scissor blade
for mediolateral
episiotomy

Scissor blade
for midline
episiotomy

Fig. 1   Mediolateral and midline (median) episiotomy.

cedure that had been a routine and standard obstetrical practice for decades in the USA and Canada. This made me wonder how and why this surgical intervention had become routine practice in the first place, why it had persisted so long despite there being apparently little evidence that it is beneficial, and why it was only now being questioned. And so my interest in episiotomy was ignited.

The chapters of this book trace the introduction, routinization, challenging and eventual decline of episiotomy in the UK and the USA. They identify and explore the medical and extra-medical factors and forces that have brought about and facilitated changes in obstetrical and midwifery thinking and use of this surgical procedure. Hopefully, by understanding how change in maternity care occurs, even in one practice, midwives, obstetricians, obstetrical nurses, antenatal teachers, childbirth activists and prospective parents wanting and attempting to change obstetric and midwifery care will be in a better position to exploit and direct the change process.

Of all obstetric interventions, episiotomy makes a particularly interesting case study because of the sheer number of women affected. This so called 'trivial' operation should be an important public health issue as it is the most frequently performed surgical procedure, after cutting the umbilical cord, and is not without sometimes serious side effects. It is performed on millions of women annually. In 1994, over 1.5 million episiotomies were performed in the USA alone and in 1985, the last year for which national data are available, another 220 000 were performed in England (personal communication with the National Center for Health Statistics; Department of Health, 1988).

The practice of episiotomy is also appealing to study because of the tremendous current international variation in the use of the operation. As Fig. 2 reveals, where only 28% of women giving birth vaginally in Belgium receive the operation, close to 100% of Japanese women and women in Central and Eastern Europe having vaginal deliveries experience an episiotomy. It is important here to note that national statistics on episiotomy use are of varying quality and, for many countries, probably represent underestimates. Furthermore, despite the well-known relationship between parity and the use of episiotomy (first-time mothers having a greater likelihood of receiving an epi-siotomy than mothers having their second or subsequent babies), national statistics on the use of episiotomy by parity have not been systematically collected by any of the countries presented in Fig. 2, with the exception of England and Sweden. The haphazard way that national statistics on episiotomy use are often collected and reported, if they happen to be collected and reported at all, is an indication of just how widely accepted the operation is in many countries and the lack of significance that has been placed on it by health officials.

I believe that the practice of episiotomy is particularly interesting, however, because of the way that the use of this operation has changed over the past 250 years. The use of episiotomy by obstetricians dates back to the eighteenth century. During the 1800s and early 1900s, the operation was seldom performed by American and British physicians.

Country	Source	Year	Episiotomy rate (% of vaginal births)
Belgium	Buekens *et al.* (1985)	1985	
Sweden*	Röckner & Olund (1991)	1989	
England	Department of Health (1988)	1985	
France	Rumeau-Rouguette *et al.* (1984)	1981	
Netherlands	Zondervan *et al.* (1995)	1990	
Finland	(E. Heminki pers. comm.)	1994	
Scotland	(S. Cole pers. comm.)		Data not collected
Canada	(D. Fowler pers. comm.)	1992	
British Columbia		1992	
Ontario		1992	
Quebec		1992	
USA	National Center for Health Statistics	1993	
Japan*	(E. Matsuyama pers. comm.)	–	
Central and Eastern Europe+	Wagner (1994); Chalmers (1995)	–	

0   20   40   60   80   100

* – episiotomy rate for primips only
‾ – routine, 95–100% for primips
+ – routine, 90–100%

Fig. 2   Episiotomy rates by selected countries.

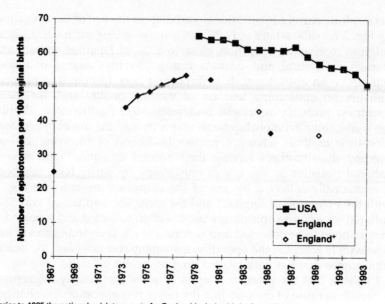

* prior to 1985 the national episiotomy rate for England includes births from Wales.
⁺ survey data, not population data (Fleissig, 1993).
Sources: Macfarlane & Mugford, 1984; Department of Health and Social Security, and Office of Population Censuses and Surveys Welsh Office, 1980, Department of Health, and Office of Population Censuses and Surveys, 1988; Kozak, 1989; National Center for Health Statistics, 1992–1995.

Fig. 3   National episiotomy rates for England* and the USA (1967–1993).

In the USA, episiotomy was increasingly adopted as a routine procedure during the 1930s and 1940s. In the UK, the restrictive use of
episiotomy persisted into the mid-1960s at which point its use began
escalating. Figure 3 graphically presents the national episiotomy rates
for the USA and England for the years 1967–1993 (the actual statistics
for each year are presented in Appendix A). As the graph shows, the
English episiotomy rate more than doubled in eleven years, climbing
from 25% of all hospital deliveries in 1967 to 53.4% in 1978. Then, over
the next seven years (1978–1985) the episiotomy rate reversed and
declined sharply from 53.4% to 36.6%, an absolute and relative
reduction of 17% and 32% respectively. In contrast to this, in the USA,
the episiotomy rate in 1979 was 65.1%, and over the next fourteen years
(1979–1993) it slowly edged down from 65.1% to 50.4%, an absolute and
relative decline of 15% and 23% respectively.

Another reason why episiotomy is interesting is that this operation,
once largely taken for granted procedure is now being questioned, not
only in the UK and USA but also in Australia (Thompson, 1987;
MacLennan, 1990), the former Czechoslovakia (Presl, 1985), Denmark
(Thranov *et al.*, 1990; Henriksen *et al.*, 1992; 1994), France (Colette,

1991), Germany (Hirsch, 1991), Italy (Mazzarella *et al.*, 1991), Japan (Chimura, 1985; Sleep, 1985), Norway (Hordnes, 1994), Quebec (Coquatrix, 1985; 1987), South Africa (Hofmeyr & Sonnendecker, 1987) and Sweden (Röckner & Olund, 1991; Röckner, 1993).

Yet one other reason for selecting episiotomy is that it is a 'low tech' or knowledge-based procedure as opposed to more 'high tech' interventions such as pharmaceuticals and medical equipment. By studying how changes have come about in the use of episiotomy, light will hopefully be shed on the reasons for the use of many low technology practices used daily by clinicians and experienced by millions of patients.

This book is essentially a cross-national case study that traces and analyses the evolution of obstetric and midwifery doctrine and use of episiotomy in the UK and the USA. While practitioners do have access to and read the world literature, this analysis is restricted primarily to the literature published in the UK , USA and Canada. This was largely a pragmatic decision relating to the cost of retrieving and translating non-English language literature.

Terminology

Before describing how the use of episiotomy has changed over time, I need to define 'innovation'. To innovate is to effect a change or make changes (*Webster's Ninth New Collegiate Dictionary*, 1991). Innovation in medicine typically refers to the adoption or abandonment of medical technology, with medical technology usually being defined as 'the set of techniques, drugs, equipment and procedures used by health care professionals in delivering medical care to individuals, and the system within which such care is delivered' (United States Congress, Office of Technology Assessment, 1976:4). I use the term innovation to refer to the generic process of change in health care technology. As health care is also provided by professionals other than physicians, I use the term health care innovation to include innovation in medicine and midwifery. In the first chapter, the term medical innovation predominates as the theories and models of innovation to date have narrowly focused on medical technology. The terms 'change' and 'innovation' are used interchangeably throughout the text.

Chapter 1

Studying the Process of Innovation in Health Care

Over the years, several theoretical models have been proposed to explain innovation in medicine or health care. The positivist model of medical innovation assumes all change is the result of scientific discoveries or thinking, and is therefore largely impervious to social forces. Contrasted with this are sociological theories of medical innovation, which are characterized by an assumption that innovation is better understood as a social activity. This chapter reviews these theories and models to explain the theoretical framework underlying the research presented in this book, and describes the methods used in conducting the research.

Ways of understanding innovation in medicine

The rational-scientific sequential model

One theory that tends to be championed by groups with authority and is often accepted by the public presents medicine as a scientifically neutral enterprise which is objective, rational and value free (Bell, 1989). This model assumes that science (i.e. scientific thinking, discoveries and research) is responsible for medical innovation. Medical technology is assumed to be the product of science and scientific thinking is assumed to determine its adoption and use.

In this positivist tradition, a number of what might be called rational-scientific sequential models have been proposed or used to explain the development of health care technology (United States Department of Health, Education and Welfare, 1976a; 1976b; United States Congress, Office of Technology Assessment, 1976; Whitted, 1981). Each of these models assumes that the development of medical technology is a relatively linear process occurring in a sequence of discrete and identifiable stages. Typically these 'ideal' models are used to trace the 'life cycle' (Banta & Thacker, 1990) or steps through which health care technology passes, as it progresses from a novel idea to its eventual adoption by care givers. Although all the rational-scientific sequential models share the same basic assumptions about the process of change in medicine, they differ in terms of the number and sequence of stages offered.

The rational-scientific sequential model receiving by far the widest exposure is the one that was offered by the Office of Technology Assessment (OTA) of the United States Congress. The OTA model of the development of medical technology was first proposed in 1976. According to this model, four general categories can be distinguished in the spectrum of activities that precede the widespread acceptance of many medical innovations. These are basic research, applied research and development, clinical testing, and diffusion (United States Congress, Office of Technology Assessment, 1976:68). A fifth stage, the widespread use of new technologies, was subsequently added (Banta & Thacker, 1979).

This model, or slight variations of it, has subsequently appeared in the medical (Banta & Thacker, 1979) and sociological literature (Banta, 1983; 1984) as well as elsewhere (Banta *et al.*, 1981; Ruby *et al.*, 1984). Furthermore, the OTA, a research agency of the US government, has used this model to explain the emergence of such medical technologies as DES (diethylstilbestrol) (Bell, 1986), as have other researchers (for example, Scheirer, 1990). (DES was a drug prescribed to millions of women to prevent miscarriage despite clinical reports that it was ineffective for this purpose. DES was also later found to cause vaginal and cervical cancer in the daughters of the women who took the drug during their pregnancies.) One of the reasons for the popularity of the OTA model in bureaucratic circles is that by conceptualizing technology development in terms of stages, formal programmes relating to each stage of development can be implemented so as to try to improve the process at each stage (Banta & Thacker, 1979).

In the following passage describing the development of medical technology, many of the major assumptions implicit in the rational-scientific sequential models of medical innovation are evident. For example, the model regards the development process as linear and unidirectional. Scientific research initiates and propels the process. As the process is based on scientific knowledge, by implication it is impervious to social forces. Furthermore, the process is considered orderly and occurs in discrete stages, with the work at each stage carried out by distinct communities.

'Adoption of a new technology by the consumer can be viewed as the final step in a long sequence of activities. First, a background or conceptual basis is laid by theoretical research and the sum of previous research. Then, basic empirical research provides a framework of knowledge about the mechanisms involved, discovers points in a natural process that are susceptible to technological intervention, and suggests strategies for technology development. Applied or mission-oriented research is then directed at applying this basic knowledge to a practical purpose and demonstrating the feasibility of the proposed technology. Once feasibility is demonstrated, engineers, entrepreneurs and developers, usually in the private sector, can develop goal-oriented programs. Prototypes are built and problems of translating the technology from the lab to the marketplace are faced. Once the manufactured item is ready, its effectiveness and efficiency can be assessed in a realistic way in industrial testing laboratories, in field tests, or in consultation with potential users. Finally, the technology is marketed and, if all goes well, it is adopted by the proper class of consumers, be they manufacturers or industries, public groups or institutions, or private individuals' (United States Congress, Office of Technology Assessment, 1976:67–8).

Despite the shortcomings of the OTA model, it made a major and enduring contribution to the study of innovation in medicine and health care by the way it defines medical technology as 'the set of techniques, drugs, equipment and procedures used by health care professionals in delivering medical care to individuals, and the system within which such care is delivered' (United States Congress, Office of Technology Assessment, 1976:4). Up to this point in time, medical technology tended to be strictly conceptualized as a thing, a physical artifact, such as a piece of equipment. The OTA definition broadened technology to include ways of doing things which might simply be skill or knowledge based.

Turning to the rational-scientific sequential models of medical technology development as a group, they suffer from several major weaknesses. Some of the problems relate to the 'rational-scientific' assumptions of these models. As identified by Bell, their greatest shortcoming in this respect is that they are 'based on a "hierarchical" model of the relationship between science and technology: scientific knowledge precedes technology development, both temporally and causally' (1989:189). For example, the very use of the expression 'applied research and development' to describe the second stage of the development process in the OTA model underscores the assumption of a direct and unique path from research to development, with research initiating the development process. Clearly, in light of the work of Maxwell (1986), Bell (1986; 1989), Valenstein (1986) and others, this assumption is untenable. To quote Maxwell (1986) who studied the role of the iron lung in the evolution of respiratory care:

'Technological change in medicine is not a single linear process, but one in which science and technology interact in complex and largely unpredictable ways' (p.24).

Another major problem with the rational-scientific sequential models of medical technology development is the assumed 'sequential' nature of the development process. While many of the models caution that the stages identified are highly idealized, basic research, applied research and development and even diffusion often progress simultaneously, not sequentially. As the OTA has pointed out, boundaries between categories are fluid and this creates problems in attempting to understand the development process when the focus is on discrete stages. As Bell (1986) has reiterated, such a model:

'...can only identify when things and procedures move from one stage to the next. Yet the development process is ongoing, and stages can be distinguished only artificially. Viewing the process as discontinuous masks the continuous streams of activities carried out by interacting communities in the development of medical technology' (p.5).

In contrast to the rational-scientific sequential models of medical technology development, sociologists and occasionally physicians have offered very different ways of understanding the process of change in medicine. These models reject the presupposition that medical innovation is primarily the product of science and suggest social forces are equally, and in some cases more important, in influencing change.

Sociological theories

Common to these social theories or models is the belief that medical innovation is a social activity; a product of human activity. For example, Bell (1986:2) who has proposed an interactive model of technology change, explicitly defines medical technology as the embodiment of human activity. Another defining characteristic of the social approach to medical innovation is the rejection of the assumption that science alone produces innovation. Instead, these models attempt to identify the extra-medical factors, such as social, political and economic forces, which give rise to medical innovation. These models simply do not assume that scientific evidence or research play a defining role in medical innovation. Sociological models of innovation include the natural history model, the political economy approach, the interactive model and the belief system approach.

The natural history model
Natural history is 'an account of an evolutionary process – a process by which not the individual, but the type evolves' (Park, 1955:36). As Bucher describes, 'It implies an unfolding course that can be analyzed in terms of phases, discernible landmarks or characteristics' (1988:132). This is an inductive approach that involves comparison of cases to

discover common traits. Existing models of innovation which can be classified under the natural history approach present change in medicine as an irrational process, with innovations being adopted before thorough testing. With its focus on the evolution of medical innovation, this approach tries to explain not only the adoption of innovations but also how they fall into disuse.

Over the years, a number of what might be considered natural histories of medical innovation have been proposed. Thinking of medical innovation as an evolving process dates back at least to the late nineteenth century. James Chadwick, a prominent Boston obstetrician of the 1880s, presents one of the earliest natural histories of medical innovation. After reviewing the obstetric and gynaecological literature of 1876–1881, he describes the 'life history' of a 'new therapeutic remedy' or 'new operation' as occurring in the following sequence of stages. First, an innovation is presented to the medical profession in the literature. Next, for reasons relating to physician self-interest, early adopters accept the innovation without evidence of its effectiveness. This is followed by more widespread acceptance until evidence mounts showing the limitations of the innovation. Then, based on the reports, positive and negative, the innovation is either adopted or rejected. Chadwick (1881) explains the process in the following way:

'An article is written, recounting the success obtained by its author in the treatment of a certain condition by a new operative method. Immediately it is tried by many practitioners, who hasten to publish their results, particularly if favorable, when they may expect to derive renown or practice from being early identified with the innovation. Articles multiply rapidly, the operation has been forced upon the attention of the whole profession; soon its charm of novelty wears off, and the number of papers would rapidly diminish, were it not that the negative or unfavorable results obtained begin to be published; the true merits of the operation are gradually reached, and finally it is either adopted or is renounced and forgotten' (p.254).

Nearly a century later, two physicians from New Orleans offered another sequential model of the process of innovation to explain the phenomenon of 'bandwagons of medicine'. Cohen and Rothschild (1979) define 'bandwagons of medicine' as the overwhelming acceptance of unproved but popular ideas, theories, practices and procedures. They describe a process which is dynamic, complex and more driven by interest-group politics than rational scientific thought. They describe 'bandwagons in medicine' thus:

'A single advocate or groups of advocates may be able to generate the necessary interest to launch the idea. Once other investigators become enthusiastic, preconceived notions blur the distinction between quality and quantity of evidence. Clinicians, laymen, the media and various interest groups all have a role in sustaining unproved ideas. Physicians often accept a new idea because it offers a simple solution to a complex problem. Pressured by their profession to keep abreast of current trends, physicians must absorb an abundance of new material. Therefore, they may read uncritically or concentrate their reading on non-technical journals and abstracts. The public, in search of a panacea, exerts further pressure on the clinician. The mass media give the idea momentum by publishing opinions, conclusions and extrapolations as data. Research foundations, government agencies and private industries may each have vested interest in the idea, endowing it with official sanction and monetary support. Once the hypothesis is generally accepted, further investigation is considered perfidious and is curbed by the reluctance to fund dissidents. Though the idea may become orthodoxy, doubts persist among an unconvinced minority, because the evidence is not conclusive. Eventually these doubts lead to a critical re-evaluation of the hypothesis. The gap left by the decline in popularity of an idea is filled either by a more viable idea or by a newly emerging bandwagon' (Cohen & Rothschild, 1979:531–2).

Within the natural history approach, McKinlay's (1981) seven stage career of a medical innovation is the most celebrated. Using the concept of a typical career as a heuristic device, McKinlay breaks down fairly complex social behaviour and political processes into a manageable form and identifies possible points of intervention. In keeping with the other natural histories of medical innovation, adoption of an innovation precedes its being evaluated for effectiveness. Once evaluated, it is often abandoned as ineffective. McKinlay's model portrays the first four stages of the career of an innovation as a political process in which a rational-scientific basis for legitimizing the adoption of the innovation is lacking. According to McKinlay, the typical career of a medical innovation is initiated with the release of a promising report. The innovation then passes through a stage of professional and organizational adoption, followed by a stage of public acceptance and state endorsement before attaining the status of a standard procedure. Only after it has become a standard practice, is it submitted to randomized controlled trials (RCTs) to evaluate its effectiveness. The two remaining stages in the career of a medical innovation are professional denunciation after RCTs reveal the innovation is not beneficial, and, finally, its erosion and discreditation.

More recently, Dixon (1990) has used a four stage model to describe the evolution of clinical policies. Clinical policies are guidelines or 'medical rules of thumb' which are developed to spell out the circumstances under which certain technologies, practices or procedures should be used. In keeping with the previous natural histories of medical innovation, Dixon (1990:201) reveals that at each stage social rather than scientific forces play a central role. He also notes that at each step errors in both reasoning and research may occur. The four stages in the evolution of clinical policies are development, diffusion, domination and disillusionment.

Bell (1986) views McKinlay's career of a medical innovation as simply another sequential model along the lines of the positivist OTA model. By doing so, however, she ignores the social activity explicit within this model. The stage model is fundamentally different from the rational-scientific sequential model in that the natural history concept identifies and directs attention to the extra-medical forces involved in the process of innovation and orients analysis to the emerging and unfolding lines of social activity. A more apt criticism of the seven stage model and natural history models in general might be that they have been presented prematurely and accepted uncritically as true descriptions of the innovation process. Perhaps there is no sequence of stages common to all changes or innovations in medicine. Alternatively there may be common stages with only certain types of innovations. For example, innovation involving pharmaceutical or biomedical equipment may be very different from innovation involving the use of only knowledge based skills.

If the complete power of the concept of natural history is to be realized, considerably more case studies must be conducted on different types of innovation to establish what, if any, common stages exist. In the meantime, using the concept of natural history or career as an analytic tool to study innovation is, as McKinlay claims, one way to break down fairly complex social behaviour and political processes. In doing this, however, one must not impose McKinlay's stages a priori, but allow stages (if there are any), to emerge from the data.

The political economy approach
A somewhat different way of understanding the process of innovation in medicine is the political economy approach. This approach offers a Marxian analysis of medical technology change and places medical innovation within the broader structural arrangements of society. Political and economic structures are assumed to determine medical innovation. Waitzkin's (1979; 1980) analysis of coronary care technology falls within this perspective. He argues that capitalist profit considerations are behind the development and growth of coronary care technology. He identifies industrial corporations, academic medical centres, private philanthropies, the health care labour force and the state as communities involved in encouraging innovation. This approach is limited, however, by its deterministic nature and complete lack of consideration of the role of science in medical innovation (Bell, 1986).

Furthermore, Waitzkin's view oversimplifies the development process as not all medical innovations involve the production of consumable products such as equipment, pharmaceuticals, supplies, etc.

Some innovations simply involve a change in the way a procedure or practice is performed – an innovation in knowledge. With these types of innovations, there may be little or no involvement of industrial corporations, private philanthropies or the state in bringing about change.

The interactive model

Building on the work of Waitzkin and others, Bell offers a complex interactive model of medical technology development. The model suggests that medical technology embodies ideas and practices. Understanding medical innovation, it follows, involves identifying which ideas and practices are embodied in medical technology and how they give rise to it (Bell, 1986). This is done by identifying communities that produce medical technology as well as their interests and ideas; locating these communities within a broad political and economic context; revealing how the communities are structurally related to each other, and showing how they resolve conflicts. As Bell explains:

'If medical technology is defined as embodied concepts and practices and if the innovation process is defined as one in which streams of activity are carried out over time by communities whose work is informed by intellectual concerns and by political, economic and social arrangements, then a number of implicit processes can be revealed and explained' (p.26).

Bell used diethylstilbestrol (DES) as a case study to demonstrate the usefulness of the interactive model in explaining medical technology development. Her analysis revealed that four communities produced DES: science, medicine, the pharmaceutical industry and the state. Within these communities she identified a number of specific groups: sex endocrinologists, elite physicians, twelve leading pharmaceutical manufacturers and the Food and Drug Administration, which communicated with each other in an ongoing way during the development of DES. She explained the interactions and communications between these groups by the politics of the New Deal period, professional networking, and attempts to make a product that was effective and safe. (The New Deal period refers to the legislative and administrative programme of President F.D. Roosevelt which was designed to promote economic recovery and social reform in the USA during the 1930s.) Bell's analysis revealed that the development of DES was facilitated by physicians during the 1930s redefining the menopause as a disease.

The belief system approach

Another social approach to studying medical innovation directs attention to the ways in which medical practice and the content of that practice are influenced by professionals' belief system/biomedical paradigm or understanding of the world. This approach can stand alone as a model for the study of medical innovation (Richards, 1975); however, it is also an important component of Bell's interactive model.

The belief system approach assumes that innovations are shaped by the belief systems or paradigms of their producers and users. Richards (1975), for example, has used this approach to explain the rapid increase in the non-medical or elective use of induction of labour in the UK during the 1970s. His analysis revealed that the apparently irrational practice of induction could be traced, in large part, to the dominant biomedical belief system of modern obstetrics in the UK. According to Richards, the increase in induction was directly related to obstetrics being a hospital based surgical speciality which tries to solve problems by active intervention. These features of the profession, he argued, encouraged a belief system which emphasized control over patients.

> 'It is this feature of obstetrics that may be the key to the process of innovation. To put the matter rather crudely, obstetrics treats the body like a complex machine and uses a series of interventionist techniques to repair faults that may develop in the machine. But given that all births (both malfunctioning and smoothly running machines) are treated obstetrically there is a constant tendency to use the repair techniques when all is going well' (Richards, 1975:598).

Other researchers have examined the relationships between the prevailing belief system within medicine and obstetrics and intervention in childbirth (Ehrenreich & English, 1979; Graham & Oakley, 1981; Katz Rothman, 1984; Rosengren & Sartell, 1986; Martin, 1989).

Theoretical framework

The theoretical framework adopted for this research blends aspects of several of the sociological models of health care innovation. I began by adopting Bell's assumption that medical innovation is the product of human activity and therefore a social as opposed to strictly scientific activity. From the natural history approach, I adopted the conceptualization of innovation as an unfolding and evolutionary process and directed my efforts toward seeking the processional character of the innovation under investigation; episiotomy. This involved documenting the phases or changes in obstetrical and midwifery thinking and use of episiotomy over time. It also directed my attention to identifying the antecedents to these changes.

From Bell's interactive model I adopted the position that innovation is complex, involving the activities of many communities occurring simultaneously. This model alerted me to the need to identify all the specific individuals and communities responsible for bringing about change as well as their interests and ideas. Being a surgical technique or knowledge based skill, the primary communities anticipated to be involved were physicians, midwives and women. Unlike other types of innovations, such as pharmaceuticals or biomedical equipment, I did not expect industry or government to have a major role in the adoption or rejection of episiotomy. The reasoning for this was that physicians in the UK and USA do not bill separately for performing or repairing the operation. This is not to say, however, that manufacturers of suture materials do not directly benefit from the routine use of episiotomy. The more episiotomies cut the more suture material sold. It has been estimated that in the USA alone this is probably worth £15 million pounds ($23 million) per year which likely accounts for suture companies taking stands at conferences and sponsoring study-days and research.

Finally, the belief system approach made me aware that innovation is influenced and moulded by the belief system of those considering any sort of change. The theoretical framework I adopted did not include the political economy approach as I did not consider that it would be very informative or useful in studying a purely knowledge based technology.

My approach to studying the process of innovation in health care was also moulded by Spector and Kitsuse's (1977) social construction of reality approach to social problems. This approach conceptualizes social problems not as a condition but as a kind of social activity. They refer to this social activity as 'claims-making'. It involves the 'protesting and complaining activities that generate awareness, policy, and response to morally offensive and objectionable conditions' (Spector, 1976:168). As Spector and Kitsuse explain about their theory:

> 'The emergence of a social problem is contingent upon the organization of activities asserting the need for eradicating, ameliorating, or otherwise changing some condition. The central problem for a theory of social problems is to account for the emergence, nature and maintenance of claims-making and responding activities' (p.76).

Drawing on Spector and Kitsuse's work, I adopted the notion of innovation in health professions as a claims-making activity, with innovation resulting from the claims-making, advocating, campaigning and questioning activities of individuals and communities intent on producing change. This notion of claims-making activity is quite compatible with Bell's interactive model. Taking the liberty of adapting Spector and Kitsuse's (1977:78) words, claims-making is always a form of interaction: a demand made by one party to another that some change be made in the way health care is practised. Also, similar to Bell's model, this approach requires identifying the individuals and groups engaged in claims-making activity, as well as the response it receives. One other similarity between my research and the social constructionist approach is that the focus of attention is on the claims-making activity not on evaluating the veracity of the claims being made. With this approach, what is most important is how the claims are made and whether they are accepted, not whether they are necessarily true.

Research methods and data

The remainder of the chapter is devoted to the research methods I used to study the process of change as it relates to obstetrics' orthodoxy about episiotomy and the operation's use. The data for this research consist primarily of documentary materials and interviews with key informants. The documentary materials are derived from diverse sources including the professional and popular literature. They are limited to the English language literature of the USA and Canada, the UK and Ireland. These materials span the period from the mid-1800s to 1995. Interviews with key informants supplement the documentary materials by providing data on the events and activities of the most recent years (roughly the period from 1970 onwards). The sources of data consulted are presented in some detail so as to provide the reader with sufficient information to judge the validity of the research findings. Additional information about the methods used can be found elsewhere (Graham, 1995).

The professional literature

The predominant sources of data, particularly for the period prior to about 1970, are medical (primarily obstetric) and midwifery (including nurse midwifery) textbooks, journals and conference proceedings. As Harold Speert (1980), an official historian of the American Gynecology Society (AGS), notes:

'The principal medium of communication in medicine has always been its "literature". Medical books and journals have served the three-fold purpose of instructing students and practitioners, recording scientific observations, and providing a forum for the expression of opinion by authors and editors' (p.124).

For these very reasons, the professional literature, as a repository of medical knowledge, may reveal why a practice was begun and continues to be performed or has been abandoned (Banta & Thacker, 1982). Journals offer a particularly rich source of data on claims-making activities. The publication of papers, editorials, commentaries and letters to the editor provide a forum for these activities. Another source of data which can provide considerable insight into the process of claims-making is scholarly discussions which take place at annual meetings of professional bodies. These data are often available in the official proceedings of conferences and meetings.

Textbooks are extremely useful for revealing current practices and thinking within a profession. Because they are intended for the instruction of novices, the practices, techniques and theories presented in textbooks tend to be ones over which there is considerable agreement. In other words, textbooks are simultaneously repositories of knowledge and orthodoxy. The comparison of consecutive editions of the same text is a fairly easy way of identifying and dating shifts in professional consensus.

Materials such as membership directories of professional associations (e.g. the *American Medical Directory*, the *Medical Directory*, the *Medical Registry*; AAOG, 1920; 1942; AGS, 1885; 1904; 1915; 1952; 1982), obituaries and organizational documents (e.g. the *Album of the Fellows of the American Gynecology Society* (Chadwick *et al.*, 1901; Broun, 1918; Keene, 1930)), are valuable sources of information on the individuals involved in bringing about change. These types of materials provide background data on an individual's training and professional credentials (e.g. specialty training, board certification, speciality association membership, academic affiliations), as well as offices held and honours received. This information is useful in providing an indication of an individual's general stature or prominence within their profession and, by implication, their potential influence on peers.

The popular literature

Prior to the 1970s, the use of episiotomy was almost exclusively a medical issue. Since that time, however, women have increasingly questioned the practice. From about 1970 onward, the consumer literature challenging the medical claims made about the use of episiotomy has been an important source of data. These data consist mainly of childbirth education books and manuals directed at expectant parents, and newspaper and women's magazine articles dealing with pregnancy, childbirth or birthing practices. I also examined the newsletters, publications and conference proceedings of childbirth organizations such as the National Association of Parents and Professionals for Safe Alternatives in Childbirth (NAPSAC), the International Childbirth Education Association (ICEA), the National Childbirth

Trust (NCT) and the Association for Improvements in the Maternity Services (AIMS).

Historical and sociological analyses

To place the episiotomy claims-making activity within its socio-historical context, I relied on what might be appropriately considered the 'childbirth literature'. This material includes histories of childbirth and the caregivers in childbirth, sociological analyses of the development and evolution of obstetrics and midwifery, and historical, sociological and anthropological analyses of the evolution of childbirth practices. This body of literature contains several perspectives on the history of childbirth: histories of the obstetric profession (Cianfrani, 1960; Speert, 1980); feminist revisions of this history (Korbin, 1966; Ehrenreich & English, 1973; 1979; Oakley, 1976; 1986; Donegan, 1978; Wertz, 1983), and a revision of this revisionist history (Shorter, 1982). I also consulted less controversial histories such as those by Donnison (1977), Scholten (1977; 1985), Wertz and Wertz (1979; 1989) and Leavitt (1986).

Interviews

For the more contemporary component of my research, I supplement the documentary research with personal interviews with twenty-three prominent individuals involved in varying aspects of childbirth research and activism. I corresponded by mail with another four key informants. All of these individuals are public figures and most were selected because of their questioning of the routine use of episiotomy during the 1970s and 1980s. They include researchers, physicians (obstetricians and family or general practitioners), midwives, childbirth activists and a women's health activist. They also include academics and a Canadian Health Department official responsible for childbirth issues. The individuals making up my key informants were David Banta, Beverley Lawrence Beech, Jean Campen (by correspondence), Iain Chalmers, Diana Elbourne, Eleanor Enkin, Murray Enkin, Caroline Flint, Doris Haire, Louise Hanvey, Robert Harrison (by correspondence), Michael House, Sally Inch, Sally Jorgenson, Sheila Kitzinger, Michael Klein, Catherine Kohler Riessman, Alison Macfarlane, Mary Renfrew, J.K. Russell (by correspondence), Jennifer Sleep, Norma Swenson, Stephen Thacker (by correspondence), Dawn Walker, Dorothy Wertz, Diony Young and Luke Zander.

For the most part, I used these interviews to verify the findings of my analysis and interpretation of the documentary data. In a number of cases, the interviews were also useful for revealing the respondents' personal interests in episiotomy, their motivation for questioning the practice, and the strategies they used to challenge the use of the practice. They also provided information on the 'behind the scenes' activities which are seldom reported in the published literature.

While not used specifically as a source of data, presentations of 'research in progress' before medical, sociological and feminist audiences provided feedback on my analysis and sometimes quite useful insights about my interpretation of the data.

Data collection methods

The documentary material

I used several strategies to locate the professional or caregiver literature on episiotomy. Initially, I conducted computerized searches of the US National Library of Medicine's database (MEDLINE). MEDLINE corresponds to the print indexes: *Index Medicus*, the *International Nursing Index* and the *Index to Dental Literature*. Information indexed on MEDLINE includes research papers, reviews of the literature, articles, editorials and letters to the editor dating from 1966. As of 1990, MEDLINE indexed articles from 3363 journals published in over 70 countries. For the professional periodical literature predating 1966, I manually searched the *Cumulative Index Medicus*. I used the search term 'episiotomy' in searching both the MEDLINE and *Cumulative Index Medicus*. 'The Index and Abstracts of the Current Literature' produced by the journal *Birth: Issues in Perinatal Care and Education* was also useful in locating episiotomy literature. This journal has indexed the periodical literature on pregnancy and childbirth since 1973.

I systematically examined the leading American and British journals in the fields of obstetrics and midwifery for references to episiotomy. These journals included:

- the *American Journal of Obstetrics and Gynecology* (from 1920 onwards), formerly the *American Journal of Obstetrics and Diseases of Women and Children* (1868–1919); this journal is known in obstetrical circles as the 'Gray Journal'. It is the world's foremost journal in obstetrics and gynaecology (Speert, 1980). It has served as the official organ of the American Gynecology Society, the American Association of Obstetricians and Gynecologists, as well as the obstetrical societies of Boston, New York, Philadelphia and many other local and regional obstetrical and gynaecological organizations.
- the *Transactions of the American Gynecological Society* (from 1868 onwards) (Chadwick, 1881).
- *Obstetrics and Gynecology* (since 1953); the speciality's most widely

read periodical in the USA (Speert, 1980). It is referred to by obstetricians as the 'Green Journal' and is the official organ of the
American College of Obstetrics and Gynecology.

- *Surgery, Gynecology and Obstetrics* (from 1905 onwards); the official
organ of the American College of Surgeons.
- *Obstetrics and Gynecology Survey* (from 1946 onwards); a journal
distinctive for the editorial comments of the editors appended to
selected abstracts of the world's literature (Speert, 1980).
- the *British Journal of Obstetrics and Gynaecology* (from 1975 onwards),
formerly the *Journal of Obstetrics and Gynaecology of the Commonwealth*
(1961–1975) and the *Journal of Obstetrics and Gynaecology of the British
Empire* (1902–1961); the official journal of the Royal College of
Obstetricians and Gynaecologists.
- the *Journal of Nurse-Midwifery*; the official journal of the American
College of Nurse Midwives.
- *Midwives Chronicle and Nursing Notes*; the official journal of the Royal
College of Midwives.
- *Midwives, Health Visitor and Community Nurse*; a popular British
midwifery journal.
- *Birth: Issues in Perinatal Care and Education* (from 1982 onwards),
formerly *Birth and the Family Journal* (1973–1981); a progressive
journal devoted to family maternity care.

I spent considerable time browsing the open and closed stacks of
McGill University's medical, nursing and history of medicine libraries,
Harvard University's Frances Countway medical library and the
library of the Royal Society of Medicine (London) to locate obstetric
and midwifery texts and monographs.

To locate the popular, consumer or lay material on episiotomy, I
manually searched *The Reader's Guide to the Periodical Literature*, *The
Magazine Index*, *The Social Science Citation Index*, *Dissertation Abstracts*,
Women Studies Abstracts, *The British Newspaper Index* and *The Times of
London Index*. For these indexes, I used the search terms 'episiotomy',
'birth', 'childbirth', 'obstetrics' and 'midwifery'.

Throughout the course of my research, whether searching for documentary material in the professional or popular/consumer literature,
I also relied on the time-honoured data collection method of following
the reference trail. I continuously traced the references cited in the
materials I retrieved.

While I was able to locate most of the material in the local medical,
history of medicine, nursing, graduate and teaching hospital libraries, I
also made good use of interlibrary loan. This service was especially
helpful in locating dissertations, obscure or highly specialized journals
and childbirth education books, and consecutive editions of medical
and midwifery textbooks. Books on childbirth preparation/education

tend to be found in public as opposed to academic libraries, making the use of interlibrary loans essential when these types of documents were to be retrieved.

Chapter 2

Nineteenth-century Challenging of the Emergency Use of Episiotomy

The obstetrical use of episiotomy has a long history. Recorded use of the procedure in the English speaking world goes back more than two-and-a-half centuries. This chapter describes the origins of episiotomy and traces the evolution of medical doctrine regarding the operation from the mid eighteenth century through the turn of the twentieth century.

A small number of 'episiotomy enthusiasts' rediscovered the operation during the latter part of the 1800s and unsuccessfully campaigned for the more widespread use of the operation. As their efforts will reveal, research and claims-making activities alone may be insufficient to produce innovation in medicine. Efforts to generate medical innovation are also moderated by social and technological factors such as the dominant belief system, the prominence of those advocating or opposing change, client demand, and the existing technology or access to it. These factors effectively neutralized the episiotomy protagonists' claims-making activities and restricted the greater use of episiotomy from the late nineteenth century through the early twentieth century.

Historical background: the first one hundred years

Although it is not known exactly when the practice of incising the perineum during childbirth began, the operation was first proposed in the literature by Sir Fielding Ould in 1742. In *Treatise of Midwifery*, the first English language textbook of obstetrics of any importance (Morton, 1954), Ould offered up incision of the perineum as a means of saving the life of the child. Ould was the second Master of the Rotunda Lying-in Hospital in Dublin and described the operation and the indication for it as follows:

'It sometimes happens, though the Labour has succeeded so well, that the Head of the Child has made its way through the Bones of the Pelvis, that it cannot however come forward, by reason of the Extraordinary Constriction of the Vagina; so that the Head, after it has passed the Bones, thrusts the Flesh and Integuments before it, as if it were contained in a Purse; in which Condition if it continues long, the Labour will become dangerous, by the Orifice of the Womb contracting about the Child's Neck; wherefore it must be dilated if possible by the Fingers, and forced over the Child's Head; if this cannot be accomplished, there must be an Incision made toward the Anus with a Pair of crooked Probe Sizars; introducing one Blade between the Head and Vagina, as far as shall be thought necessary for the present Purpose, and the Business is done at one Pinch, by which the whole Body will easily come forth.' (Parvin citing Ould, 1882:151–2)

Over the next hundred years or so, the operation remained relatively obscure in the English speaking world, although numerous European physicians experimented with it. During the first half of the nineteenth century, these physicians proposed several modifications or variations to Ould's method. They also tended to look on episiotomy as more a means of preventing a spontaneous perineal laceration or rupture than a technique for simply widening the birth canal in order to facilitate an extremely difficult birth.

It appears that the first physician to actually report performing perineal incision was G. Ph. Michaelis from Harburg, Germany. In work published in 1810, Michaelis described how on 17 April 1799 he used a Pott's bistoury to enlarge a three-quarter of an inch perineal tear by about an inch, whereupon the birth continued spontaneously without further tearing (David, 1993).

In 1820, in a textbook on the use of mechanical aids for childbirth, Ritgen suggested making multiple superficial incisions around the vaginal orifice as an effective method of protecting the perineum from rupture (David, 1993).

In France, Professor Dubois is credited with being the first to suggest making an oblique incision in the perineum in 1847 (Nugent, 1935). This practice is known today as mediolateral episiotomy. In 1850 and 1852, Eichelberg and Scanzoni recommended lateral and bilateral episiotomy (the making of lateral incisions perpendicular to the vaginal orifice) (Stahl, 1895).

Despite the numerous methods advanced for incising the perineum during the first half of the nineteenth century, there is little indication that the operation ever gained wide acceptance among physicians. As one late nineteenth century physician remarked about Michaelis' 1810 suggestion that median incision prevented rupture of the perineum, 'the recommendation did not meet with favour' (Broomall, 1878:517). Indeed, there was so little general interest in the operation that it went unnamed until 1857 when Carl Braun of Vienna suggested the term 'episiotomy' which literally means cutting of the vulva or pubic area. Braun himself had little use for the operation and condemned it as inadvisable and unnecessary (Nugent, 1935).

In the USA and Canada the situation was much the same. Incision of the perineum was seldom, if ever, performed. The first reported use of the operation was by a Virginian surgeon who performed it on 2 December 1851 (Schmidt, 1959). Writing about the case the following year in *The Stethoscope and Virginia Gazette,* the surgeon remarked:

'When this was done by me I was not aware of its having been done before, and was really afraid that my professional brethren would condemn me...'
(Taliaferro cited by Longo, 1976:115).

Episiotomy as a 'last resort'

Between the 1870s and the second decade of the twentieth century, the operation of episiotomy became increasingly accepted as an operation of last resort in cases where the perineum was thought to be at extreme risk of rupturing. During these years, a growing number of distinguished obstetricians in the USA, England, Scotland and Ireland cautiously began condoning the use of episiotomy as an operation of desperation. In their textbooks and published monographs on management of the perineum during childbirth, these leading obstetrical authorities emphasized that the operation was to be reserved for those relatively few abnormal or extremely difficult cases where the then currently accepted non-surgical methods of preventing a severe perineal laceration seemed unlikely to be effective.

These physicians' approbation of the emergency use of episiotomy rested primarily on their belief that the operation offered a means of controlling the extent and location of an impending laceration. They reasoned that if a laceration seemed inevitable, by performing an episiotomy the physician could choose the location and depth of the wound, something not thought possible with a spontaneous laceration. The obstetric authorities advised their colleagues that by performing an episiotomy they could thereby save the anal sphincter by diverting an impending laceration away from it. Some also suggested an incised perineum healed as well as, or better than, a spontaneous laceration. Others, however, disputed this view, believing instead that spontaneous lacerations healed just as well as incised trauma and without complication.

The following sample of quotations from Simpson, Madden and Lusk is illustrative of what some of the most influential English speaking obstetrical authorities of the late nineteenth and early twentieth century were saying about the use of episiotomy.

Sir James Young Simpson, one of the best-known obstetricians of his day, is noted for his discovery and use of obstetrical anaesthesia (chloroform) for which he received a baronetcy from Queen Victoria in

1866 (Graham, 1960:256). He is also claimed by some biographers as the chief individual responsible for laying the foundation of gynaecology as a separate branch of medicine (Thoms, 1935). Concerning prevention of a 'central perineal laceration', Simpson advises first employing the 'common methodic manual support of the perineum' followed by delivery of the head by forceps, and then:

> '...lateral incisions, if absolutely necessary, of the interior edge of the perineum, for in this, it is, I believe, better practice to make one or two slight cuts on either side of the fourchette, so as to regulate the site and direction of the lacerations that must occur, rather than leave their form and their character to mere chance alone. It is always an indefinitely more important matter to save the sphincter of the anus than the sphincter of the vagina' (Simpson, 1871:594–5).

Thomas More Madden, a member of the Royal College of Surgeons, Examiner in Midwifery and Diseases of Women and Children, Queen's University, Ireland, and Ex-Assistant Physician at the Rotunda Lying-in Hospital, Dublin, endorsed the use of episiotomy in a paper published in the first medical speciality journal devoted to the field of obstetrics and gynaecology, the *American Journal of Obstetrics and Diseases of Women and Children*. In his article entitled 'On Laceration of the Perinaeum, Sphincter Ani, and Recto-vaginal Septum – Their Prevention and Surgical Treatment', Madden advises:

> 'When this accident [perineal laceration] appears otherwise inevitable, it may sometimes be obviated by incising the perinaeum in such a manner as to afford a sufficient passage for the child, and at the same time, protect the mother from the possibility of a recto-vaginal laceration.... It has recently been proposed, in cases of impending laceration of the perinaeum during labor, that an incision should be made through the thin, expanded structures so as to relieve the existing tension. I have put this suggestion into practice in several cases with great advantage, as the perinaeum was thereby generally saved from laceration, which had previously appeared inevitable. Moreover, the wound thus made was limited to the extent of the incision, and generally healed within a few days without any special treatment. I do not recommend this measure, however, excepting in those comparatively very rare cases in which well-directed manual support would fail to protect the perinaeum' (Madden, 1872:57–8).

The last sample quotation comes from the American textbook *The Science and Art of Midwifery* by Lusk. William Lusk was Professor of Obstetrics and Diseases of Women and Children and of Clinical Midwifery at Bellevue Hospital Medical College, New York, and a founder (1876), Vice-President (1889) and President (1894) of the AGS (Chadwick *et al.*, 1901). His textbook is considered one of the two major American obstetrical texts of the latter part of the nineteenth century

(Speert, 1980). Under the heading 'Preservation of the Perineum', Lusk counsels:

> 'When, in the judgment of the physician, rupture of the perinaeum seems inevitable, he is justified in making lateral incisions through the vulva to relieve the strain upon the recto-vaginal septum. To this operation the term episiotomy is applied. By it not only is the danger of deep laceration through the sphincter ani prevented, but, owing to their eligible position, the wounds themselves are capable of closing spontaneously; whereas, when laceration follows the raphe, the retraction of the transversi perinaei muscles causes a gaping place which interferes with immediate union. As, however, every wound surface is a source of danger in childbed, episiotomy should never be performed so long as hope exists of otherwise preserving the perinaeum. It is essentially the operation of young practitioners, the occasion for its employment diminishing in frequency with increasing experience' (Lusk, 1884:210).

The above discussion of episiotomy remained unchanged in the subsequent 1885 and 1895 editions of Lusk's textbook.

The use of episiotomy as a measure of last resort was also acknowledged or advocated by numerous other well-known physicians of the day. Many of these physicians held professorships at some of the most prestigious medical schools and several were authors of popular obstetrical textbooks. They included

Fordyce Barker (1874), Professor of Clinical Midwifery and Diseases of Women at Bellevue Hospital Medical College, New York;
Montrose Pallen (1876), Professor of Gynecology at the University of New York;
Henry Garrigues (1880), Professor of Obstetrics in the Postgraduate Medical Schools and Hospital of New York;
William Playfair, (1882; 1885; 1889; 1898), Professor of Obstetric Medicine at King's College, London;
Theophilus Parvin (1882; 1890; 1895), Professor of Obstetrics and Diseases of Women and Children at the Indianapolis College of Physicians and Surgeons;
Thad Reamy (1885), Professor of Obstetrics, Clinical Midwifery and Diseases of Women and Children at the Medical College of Ohio;
Barton Cooke Hirst (1902), Professor of Obstetrics at the University of Pennsylvania;
J. Chalmers Cameron (1903), Professor of Obstetrics and Disease of Infancy at McGill University, Montreal;
James Clifton Edgar (1903; 1904; 1913), Professor of Obstetrics and Clinical Midwifery at Cornell Medical College, New York;
J. Clarence Webster (1903), Professor of Obstetrics and Gynecology, Rush Medical College, University of Chicago;

Henry Jellett (1905), Gynaecologist and Obstetrician to Dr Stevens' Hospital, Dublin;
Alfred Galabin, Late Fellow of Trinity College, Cambridge University and George Blacker, Fellow of the University College, London (Galabin & Blacker, 1910);
Thomas Watts Eden (1911), Examiner in Midwifery and Diseases of Women at the University of Oxford and the Royal Army Medical College, Aldershot;
Robert Johnstone (1913), Assistant to the Professor of Midwifery, University of Edinburgh;
and J. W. Ballentyne (1919), Lecturer on Midwifery and Gynaecology, School of Medicine of the Royal College of Surgeons' Hall, Edinburgh.

That the men endorsing the use of episiotomy as a last resort were in fact leading obstetrical authorities is also evidenced by their membership of professional bodies. All were members of the prestigious AGS or the Royal Colleges of Physicians and Surgeons (England, Scotland and Ireland). The AGS is the oldest national gynaecological society in the world (founded in 1867). Membership of it has been referred to as 'an accolade of the highest order' (Beacham, 1953:117). Initially, membership was restricted to 60 Fellows. Candidates had to be nominated by the Council and required a two-thirds affirmative vote of all the Fellows to be accepted. Since that time, membership has continued to be coveted. In 1968 the AGS passed a resolution increasing membership to a maximum of 120 Fellows, although the actual number of Fellows did not reach 100 until 1972 (Speert, 1980).

At the time of their endorsement of the emergency use of episiotomy, eight American obstetricians were Fellows of the AGS: three were founding members (Barker, Lusk and Parvin); another four were elected Fellows (Garrigues, 1877; Reamy, 1877; Hirst, 1889; Edgar, 1893); and one an Honorary Fellow (Webster, 1898). Parvin and Reamy had been elected to the Council of the AGS (1876–77 and 1883 respectively) and Reamy had served as Vice-President in 1881. In the ensuing years, five of these men were eventually elected President of the AGS (Barker, 1876; 1877; Reamy, 1886; Parvin, 1893; Lusk, 1894; Hirst, 1924;), five served as Vice-President (Parvin, 1883; 1886; Lusk, 1889; Garrigues, 1897; Edgar, 1907; Hirst, 1922), two served on Council (Garrigues, 1882; Barker, 1883) and two were elected Honorary Fellows (Garrigues, 1901; Cameron, 1910).

Physicians from England, Scotland and Ireland who favoured last resort use of episiotomy were also prominent as evidenced by their credentials. Prior to the formation of the College of Obstetricians and Gynaecologists, London in 1929 (later becoming the Royal College), membership of the Royal Colleges of Physicians and Surgeons indicated prominence within the profession. Of all the English, Scottish and Irish physicians, almost all were either Fellows of the Royal College of Physicians of London (Blacker, Eden and Galabin), the Royal College of Physicians of Edinburgh (Ballentyne), the Royal College of Surgeons of Edinburgh (Blacker, Eden and Johnstone), the Royal College of Physicians of Ireland (Jellett), or a Member of the Royal College of Surgeons of Ireland (Madden). Two physicians practising in Canada and the USA also belonged to the Royal Colleges of Physicians. Cameron was a Member of the Royal College of Physicians of London and Webster was a Fellow of the Royal College of Physicians of Edinburgh.

The rediscovery of episiotomy and late nineteenth-century pleas for its liberal use

While the distinguished obstetric authorities of the latter part of the nineteenth century were endorsing the use of episiotomy strictly as an emergency operation, a small number of mostly American physicians attempted to broaden the indications for episiotomy by issuing pleas that the operation be performed considerably more frequently. These physicians, who are best described as episiotomy protagonists or enthusiasts, published for the first time ever papers devoted entirely to the issue of episiotomy. These pleas for the liberal use of episiotomy appeared in the *American Journal of Obstetrics and Diseases of Women and Children* (Broomall, 1878; Manton, 1885), *Archiv für Gynäkologie* (Credé & Colpe, 1884), the *New York Medical Journal* (Wilcox, 1885), the *Brooklyn Medical Journal* (Jewett, 1890), and the *Annals of Gynaecology and Paediatry* (Stahl, 1895).

Believing that perineal incision did not seem to be receiving 'at the hand of English and American writers on the subject of obstetrics, the attention its merits entitle it' (Wilcox, 1885:176), the episiotomy enthusiasts set out to popularize the operation by making several claims about the benefits of the operation. Some repeated the already familiar belief that episiotomy offered physicians some control over the extent and location of a perineal rupture. For example, Broomall (1878) and Wilcox (1885) emphasized that the operation provided a method of managing extremely unpredictable perineal lacerations. The following quotation illustrates how important the issue of control over perineal lacerations was to these episiotomy protagonists.

'Granting that a laceration is inevitable, the operation removes it from the median line and locates it in the exact position chosen by the *accoucheur*. This avoids the danger of a laceration through the sphincter ani, and also relieves the strain upon the recto-vaginal septum, preventing a central rupture.... Also ... episiotomy limits the extent of the lesion...'(Wilcox, 1885:177-8).

In some cases, episiotomy enthusiasts went even further and proposed that the operation actually prevented perineal lacerations altogether, or reduced them to an absolute minimum (Credé & Colpe, 1884; Wilcox, 1885; Manton, 1885; Jewett, 1890). Another claim issued by Credé and Colpe (1884) and then Manton (1885) was that the operation shortened labour, thereby diminishing the suffering of the mother during a prolonged and painful labour.

Jewett (1890) and Stahl (1895) advocated the greater use of episiotomy for yet another reason. They believed that an episiotomy followed by repair restored the perineum to its original integrity, something not thought to happen with spontaneous lacerations.

'I have been frequently struck with the depth and solidity of the perineal body after a typical episiotomy which has been sutured and healed. The tonicity of the pelvic floor is in marked contrast with that which usually follows the immediate suture of a deeply lacerated perineum' (Jewett, 1890:708).

Lastly, Stahl (1895) repeated Ould's assertion that episiotomy saved the lives of infants:

'... episiotomy is an instrument, *par excellence*, aiding as no other instrument in the preservation of life and body both in the foetal and maternal, and as I grow in obstetrics ... I am glad to know that there is so effectual and yet simple an instrument as central episiotomy at my command. In private practice it has often assisted me in saving the life of the foetus and always in preserving the perineal body and other parts of the soft outlet' (Stahl, 1895:676).

Episiotomy protagonists' claims-making activities and the use of evidence

As with the endorsement of the emergency use of episiotomy which rested entirely on obstetrical authorities' own positive clinical experiences with the operation, much of the evidence offered by the episiotomy protagonists in support of the more frequent use of episiotomy also took the form of personal testimonials. Stahl's quotation above of how episiotomy had 'often assisted' him 'in saving the life of the foetus and always in preserving the perineal body and other parts of the soft outlet' is an example of this strategy.

Some episiotomy protagonists, however, argued for their position in a manner that had no precedent. They provided what should have been considered at the time fairly sophisticated statistical evidence in support of their claims. These episiotomy enthusiasts were essentially making evidence-based recommendations for obstetrical practice well before Abraham Flexner made the notion of scientific medicine fashionable in 1910. Broomall (1878:526–7), for example, reported on a series of 212 patients, of which 56 had received an episiotomy. In support of her observations, she provided a table listing the 56 episiotomy cases along with data collected on nearly a dozen characteristics of the mother (e.g. age, number of pregnancies, number of vulva incisions, duration of the second stage, etc.) and half-a-dozen characteristics of the infant (e.g. presentation and position of the fetus, birthweight, occipito-frontal diameter, etc.). Based on these data she concluded that in nearly all the cases episiotomy saved the perineum, was not attended by haemorrhage, healed readily, did not complicate the lying-in and was painless as 'patients complain of no suffering' (Broomall, 1878:524).

Relying even more heavily on research, Credé and Colpe (1884) presented an analysis of 1000 consecutive primiparous cases from their clinic in Leipsic, Germany to support their contention that episiotomy prevented perineal lacerations. Comparing the percentage of episiotomies and ruptures of five successive birth assistants, Credé and Colpe reported that the occurrence of lacerations diminished in direct proportion to the frequency with which perineal incisions were performed. Crede and Colpe provided a table to support their conclusion.

Attempting to overcome expected physician resistance to their episiotomy pleas, Wilcox and Manton used Credé and Colpe's data to statistically refute three of the risks commonly attributed to the operation: that incising the perineum did not always prevent a perineal laceration, that the episiotomy incision often became infected, and that an episiotomy lengthened the lying-in period. Addressing the concern that perineal lacerations, or ruptures, occurred in spite of performing an episiotomy, Manton showed this was not a common occurrence. He noted that of Credé's 1000 cases, there were 259 episiotomies (25.9%) and only 29 ruptures in spite of incision (2.9%) compared with 104 spontaneous ruptures (10.4%).

To deal with the argument that episiotomy might increase chances of infection and lengthen the lying-in period, both Manton and Wilcox performed essentially an uncontrolled comparison. They statistically compared women who received an episiotomy with those who remained intact or suffered a perineal laceration. The following passage provides one example of how Wilcox skilfully used data to reject these anticipated criticisms of the operation.

'One of the strongest objections to this operation has been that it offers a point for general infection. That infection more frequently results from coincident tears in the vagina or cervix is stated above; the observations in the Leipsic clinic confirm this view, there being a difference of only three-tenths of one per cent in cases of puerperal fever in patients suffering from injured perinaeum over those occurring when the perinaeum was intact. Indeed among fatal cases of puerperal fever, two-hundredths of one per cent represents the difference of death rate in favor of injured perinaea, conclusively showing that the condition of the perinaeum had nothing to do with either mild or severe cases of puerperal fever. Nor are figures wanting to show that this operation shortens the time of convalescence, for the cases of episiotomy that remained over fourteen days were twenty-one and two-tenths per cent; cases of ruptured perinaeum remaining over the above time, twenty-six and nine-tenths per cent; cases of rupture in spite of episiotomy remaining over the same time were thirty-one per cent of the whole number' (Wilcox, 1885:179).

Manton dealt with this issue by observing the following:

'In 2000 cases examined by Credé, there were records of 33 deaths. Autopsy showed 19 of these to be due to septic infection; the other 14 cases were caused by eclampsia, uterine rupture and intercurrent diseases. Of the 19 septic cases, 15 were found in 1572 cases where the perineum was *intact* – a percentage of 0.954; while only 4 died who had perineal laceration – a percentage of 0.934, a scarcely appreciable difference. This would seem to indicate that the chances for infection are about equal, whether episiotomy is done or not' (Manton, 1885:233).

The episiotomy enthusiasts also appreciated that pronouncements of prominent authorities about not using episiotomy could effectively undermine the success of their pleas for episiotomy. As the following passage reveals, the episiotomy protagonists intentionally adopted the strategy of using evidence to challenge the 'opinions' of these great men.

'But when so distinguished an *accoucheur* as Dr Playfair says of episiotomy that he "questions if it is likely to be of use", we believe that the operation has not been done sufficiently in the lying-in wards of King's College Hospital to prove its efficacy. One hesitates to criticise the opinions of men who are known to the world as Nestors in their individual specialties, and yet investigation often tends to overthrow such opinions, and place in their stead facts, which in their turn must also pass through the fire' (Manton, 1885:226).

Despite the apparent statistical evidence supporting their claims and refuting common objections to the operation, the episiotomy enthusiasts' pleas appear to have had little effect on the medical establishment. In the opinion of one late nineteenth century American physician, episiotomy was 'almost wholly neglected by practitioners' (Jewett, 1890:708). The majority of physicians, this writer believed, probably never performed the operation at all.

By the second decade of the twentieth century, there is strong evidence that the weight of professional opinion had yet to be swayed by the arguments of the episiotomy enthusiasts. Episiotomy continued to be considered a measure of last resort for preventing a severe perineal laceration. A unique mail survey of ten 'prominent' American obstetricians conducted in 1915 reveals that six admitted the operation was a useful 'safety measure' for avoiding perineal laceration and all but two performed episiotomy (Rothschild, 1915). However, nine out of the ten obstetricians reported 'rarely', if ever, performing the operation or using it in less than 5% of their deliveries.

Consensus about the emergency use of episiotomy remained strong as confirmed by the influential Scottish physician J.W. Ballentyne. In a 1919 paper on methods of protecting the perineum during childbirth, Ballentyne, the so-called 'founding father' of British antenatal care (Oakley, 1986), reviewed nine of the leading early twentieth century American, English, Scottish and Irish obstetrical and midwifery texts. He spoke for physicians on both sides of the Atlantic when he concluded that now '... most admit its value in exceptional cases'. Personally endorsing the operation, Ballentyne writes:

'The writer of this critical summary is ... very favourably impressed with the value of episiotomy, especially in primipara, and he has used it with increasing frequency in late years. He believes he has often saved the median line by its employment' (Ballentyne, 1919; 409).

In keeping with the majority of obstetric authorities he had consulted, Ballentyne also noted that he was only 'ready to admit the propriety of such a surgical procedure in desperate cases' (p.411).

Additional confirmation exists that the episiotomy protagonists were unsuccessful in overcoming the obstetrical authorities' limited endorsements of episiotomy. With the exception of Garrigues (1880), who made passing reference to Broomall's paper (1878), the pleas of the episiotomy protagonists failed to be acknowledged in the writings of the obstetrical authorities of the day.

Barriers to innovation: factors preventing the widespread use of episiotomy

To understand the process of medical innovation, it is important to consider not only factors responsible for change but also the forces serving to prevent it. The failure of the episiotomy protagonists resulted from a number of factors including:

- the prevalent notion of birth as a physiological process not requiring surgical intervention;

- anticipated patient resistance;
- the unpredictable nature of perineal lacerations;
- risks commonly attributed to the operation; and
- the lack of prominence of most of the episiotomy enthusiasts (or conversely the influence of authorities opposing the widespread use of episiotomy).

The natural law of the perineum

Probably the most important factor that impeded the more liberal use of episiotomy as proposed by the episiotomy protagonists during the later part of the nineteenth century was the dominant belief system in obstetrics at the time. During the late 1800s, childbirth was conceptualized as an essentially normal or physiological process. This view also applied to the functioning of the perineum during birth. Most physicians of the day accepted what was known as the 'natural law: ... normally every perineum will properly distend to allow the exit of the child, leaving all the tissues intact' (Dewees, 1889:841). The following passages from three leading obstetrical authorities explain the 'natural law' as it pertained to the perineum.

The first from 1871 is offered by William Goodell, who at the time was Clinical Lecturer on Diseases of Women and Children at the University of Pennsylvania. Goodell was later appointed Clinical Professor of the Diseases of Women and Children, University of Pennsylvania, one of the first chairs in gynaecology in the USA (Speert, 1980). He was to become a founder and President of the Philadelphia Medical Society and a founder and Vice-President of the AGS. The second passage from 1880 is by Henry Garrigues, Professor of Obstetrics in the Postgraduate Medical School and Hospital in New York and Fellow of the AGS. The final passage from 1904 is by Ely Van de Warker, Surgeon to the Central New York Hospital for Women and a founder and former-President (1901) of the AGS.

'Is it not marvelous, that in the management of the only stage of labour which appeals to more than one of the five senses of the physician – those of sight and touch – there is a greater diversity of opinion than in that of any other stage? Is not this fact a strong argument that the perineum was made to take care of itself, and not to be supported? "We cannot" – writes Senca – "complain of the malignity of nature". "Am I to believe" – asks Leishman – "that nature, after making such admirable provision for the earlier stages of labour, bungles matters to such an extent at the end, as to render the aid of the obstetrician in every case necessary to remedy a mechanical deficiency!"

When one sees, for the first time, the maternal soft parts stretched out to a diaphanous thinness by the presenting part of the child, to all appearances just upon the point of cracking open, the impulse to place the hand upon the bulging flesh becomes almost an instinct. We must not, however, forget that these tissues are not only elastic, but living and sentient; and – what is still greater weight – that the process of labour is a strictly physiological act. Nature in all her operations intends to adapt means to ends, and the perineum was certainly not created to be torn, unless shored up by the hand of the physician' (Goodell, 1871:71).

'...the physician is the servant, not the master, of Nature. Nature always leads the greatest diameter of the child through the greatest diameter of the maternal parts, and attains this end by those wonderful turnings and adaptations, the particulars of which are not even fully understood' (Garrigues, 1880:249).

'The normal elasticity of the perineum should not be interfered with. The perineum has the capacity to stretch, to elongate, instead of tear. It seems to be the natural endowment of the perineum if it is not carried beyond the breaking point' (Van de Warker, 1904:227).

As long as the obstetrical belief system supported the view that Nature ensured the proper distension of the perineum during childbirth, physicians were philosophically discouraged from surgically intervening in the second stage of labour. That is, unless confronted by an extremely abnormal or emergency situation; the very conditions under which obstetrical authorities were sanctioning the use of episiotomy. Under normal conditions, which were thought to apply to the vast majority of births, there was simply no theoretical justification for performing an episiotomy regardless of the claims the episiotomy protagonists were making. Given this generalized belief in the 'natural law', the episiotomy protagonists' pleas for the more liberal use of perineal incision went, not surprisingly, unheeded.

Anticipated patient resistance

Physicians may have also been reluctant to adopt the liberal use of episiotomy for a reason more directly related to self interest. At this time, women also believed that childbirth was a physiologic process which did not require physician intervention in most cases. Midwives, who did not perform episiotomy, attended the vast majority of American births prior to the turn of the twentieth century. Physicians may have been unwilling to offend the minority of women who secured their services during childbirth by performing an unwanted and unappreciated episiotomy. The following statement made as late as the 1920s by a rural physician reflects this fear.

'New ideas and methods are being brought to our notice almost every day, but it is well for the man and woman in private practice to exercise considerable caution in the use of new and untried methods. We have not only the welfare of the mother and child to consider, but we must give a little attention to our professional reputations in the community.... We who are in private practice must work under the more or less close scrutiny of the patient's relatives, who all too often have been brought up in the belief that nature should be allowed to take her course unaided and that interference of any sort is flying in the face of Providence. Most patients will forgive a doctor for almost any degree of laceration if he explains the conditions that caused it and makes an honest attempt at repair, but very few of them fail to be critical of an episiotomy that fails to heal readily. No matter how urgently it was indicated the family are apt to show resentment' (Neal, 1923:292).

Leavitt (1986:152) cites a comment made in 1903 by another physician (Whery) which indicates that physicians may have been reluctant to perform the operation because patients objected to the procedure.

'Episiotomy has often been recommended, but it is only a substitution of certainty of laceration for an uncertain laceration. The patient, if she were conscious, would object to the laceration.'

The unpredictability of perineal lacerations

On a more practical level, the very nature of perineal lacerations also discouraged the more frequent use of perineal incision. During the nineteenth century, episiotomy enthusiasts promoted episiotomy as a means of managing and even preventing perineal lacerations. On the other hand, the fact that lacerations were not predictable also meant a physician could never know with certainty when an episiotomy was absolutely necessary. For example, on predicting the occurrence of perineal laceration during childbirth, Parvin, in his widely adopted American textbook *The Science and Art of Obstetrics*, writes:

'The late Dr McClintock stated that he had so often seen the perineum escape laceration where this accident seemed inevitable, he was led to doubt the possibility of recognizing the cases where incision is an absolute necessity. In view of this statement one might require conditions for episiotomy similar to those which Coleridge did for the Caesarean operation: "I think there are only two things wanting to justify a surgeon in performing the Caesarean operation: first, that he should possess infallible knowledge of his art; and, secondly, that he should be infallibly certain that he is infallible"' (Parvin, 1882:152–3).

As late as 1910, Galabin and Blacker, in the seventh edition of their British text *The Practice of Midwifery*, were still pointing out that lacerations were unpredictable, making the decision to perform an episiotomy extremely difficult.

'The plan recommended by some, namely, to perform *episeiotomy* [sic] ... in order to avoid a central laceration, is not generally desirable. For it is never possible to be certain when, and to what extent, a laceration is inevitable...' (Galabin & Blacker, 1910:648).

Being uncertain as to when an episiotomy was necessary also meant that performing the operation required the physician to abandon any hope of delivering the woman intact, the only outcome for both the woman and the doctor that was in accordance with the 'natural law'. When this dilemma is considered within the context in which physicians were attending women in childbirth, the decision to remain restrictive in the use of episiotomy is quite understandable. Prior to 1900, over 95% of births in the USA and Canada took place at home (Wertz & Wertz, 1979). During homebirths, physicians worked under varying conditions. They often complained of there being insufficient light and little assistance other than a relative or neighbour. Under these circumstances, performing an unnecessary episiotomy and inflicting a wound that might not have otherwise occurred was not a gamble most physicians were willing to take.

Risks attributed to the operation and lack of necessary supporting technology to carry out the procedure

Aside from the issue of not knowing when an episiotomy was necessary, apprehension about the side effects of episiotomy also discouraged the liberal use of the operation. The most frequently mentioned concerns about the risks of the operation were that it would be painful, the incision might not heal well or become the site of infection. These fears reflected limitations in the existing technology necessary to safely carry out perineal incision.

For example, the use of episiotomy during this period was probably impeded by limitations in the technique of episiotomy repair (the method of suturing, type of suture material, etc.). Episiotomy protagonists advised incising the perineum, yet neglected to discuss seriously how the wound should be closed. It was around this same time that a typical treatment for a spontaneous perineal laceration was to bind the woman's legs together for several weeks until the wound healed. Furthermore, the use of local anaesthesia to render episiotomy repair painless had yet to be proposed. In fact, the suggestion that episiotomy incisions should even be sutured first appeared in the published literature in 1876 (Broomall, 1878).

Along the same lines, prior to the age of Listerism in the 1880s, fears that the incision could become the site of infection (puerperal fever) was a justifiable concern as well. Had surgical technology been refined to a level where the alleged benefits of performing an episiotomy outweighed the perceived risks, protagonists' pleas might have been more successful in convincing physicians to make use of the procedure in non-emergency situations.

The importance of professional stature

Lastly, in contrast to the influential obstetrical authorities who endorsed the natural law of the perineum and the emergency use of episiotomy, most of the episiotomy protagonists lacked the prominence needed to counteract the weight of obstetrical opinion. As the eminent Samuel Gross, Emeritus Professor of Surgery, Jefferson Medical College, Philadelphia and founder and first president of the American Surgical Association, noted, 'We are too apt, as a profession, to be influenced by prejudice, especially when it is backed by great authority' (1884:342).

With two exceptions, the physicians campaigning for the liberal use of episiotomy were early in their careers and quite unknown. For example, one was a woman physician who held the position of Resident Physician at the Woman's Hospital in Philadelphia (Anna Broomall). As an indication of Broomall's status within obstetrics, her paper promoting a more liberal approach to episiotomy was delivered before the Obstetrical Society of Philadelphia not by her but by her mentor, Dr Albert Smith. Women were excluded from addressing this elite society or becoming a member of it. Another proponent, Walter Manton, had recently returned to the USA from spending three years abroad studying medicine in Europe and England, indicating that he was earlier in his medical career and would not have been widely known. Biographical information on Reynold Wilcox and Frank Stahl during this period is virtually non-existent, suggesting that both lacked prominence and influence.

The two of the episiotomy protagonists who can be counted among the obstetric authorities of the day were Chas Jewett and Carl Credé. At the time of his plea for episiotomy, Jewett was Professor of Obstetrics and Diseases of Women at Long Island College Hospital, New York and a Fellow of the AGS. He was also an ex-president of the Medical Society of the County of Kings, New York (1878–80). Of all the episiotomy protagonists of the late nineteenth century, Credé would have been most widely known. Credé, a German physician, is famous for introducing the prophylactic use of silver nitrate drops for infantile blindness, and a method of manual extraction of the placenta, both of which he proposed around the same time as routine use of episiotomy. Apparently, Jewett and Credé's reputations were insufficient to convince the profession to adopt the liberal use of episiotomy.

Chapter 3

The American Crusade for Prophylactic Episiotomy

The changing use of episiotomy

During the 1930s, discussions in the literature concerning episiotomy suggest that the operation was no longer being considered strictly an emergency procedure and was beginning to be performed quite frequently. In 1937, papers written by two fairly prominent physicians from different parts of the USA appeared back-to-back in the *American Journal of Surgery*, revealing the growing acceptance of the operation. In the first paper, Howard Taylor, an Associate Professor of Obstetrics and Gynecology at the New York University College of Medicine, Fellow of both the AGS and the American College of Surgeons, and Diplomat of the newly created American Board of Obstetrics and Gynecology, reports:

'After discussions dating back a century or more and continuing till within a few years ago, little argument now exists as to the justifiable inclusion of episiotomy among the valuable surgical procedures in obstetrics' (1937:403).

In the second paper, Willard Cooke, Professor of Obstetrics at the University of Texas, Diplomat of the American Board of Obstetrics and Gynecology, and Fellow of both the AGS and American Association of Obstetricians, Gynecologists and Abdominal Surgeons, declares:

'...episiotomy as a routine measure in all cases...is done by a great many of the best obstetricians. The procedure is unnecessary in approximately 10 per cent of primipara and in a much higher percentage of multipara...' (1937:416).

Similar statements about the use of episiotomy were also being echoed at obstetrical meetings around the country. For example, during a discussion of a paper presented before the Obstetrical and Gynecological Section of the California Medical Association in May 1937, one discussant stated 'episiotomy as a routine procedure is the rule rather than the exception in the practice of modern obstetrics'

(McCausland, 1938:178). The following year, Martin Diethelm, a Diplomat of the American Board of Obstetrics and Fellow of the American College of Surgeons, proclaimed before the Section on Obstetrics and Gynecology of the Ohio State Medical Association, 'episiotomy is today of all obstetric surgery the most frequently performed' (Diethelm, 1938:1107).

By 1950, the routine use of episiotomy was so well entrenched as standard obstetrical practice in the USA that the tenth edition of *Williams Obstetrics*, reported, 'Except for cutting and tying the umbilical cord, episiotomy is the most common operation in obstetrics' (Eastman, 1950:410).

Table 3.1 lists episiotomy rates reported by a number of individual institutions and physicians in the USA and Canada between the 1930s and 1970s. The rates are selective and may not be representative of the national picture. However, they do confirm that for the most part the operation was frequently performed during these years. During the 1930s and 1940s, with a few exceptions (Johns Hopkins University in 1930 and the Chicago Lying-In Center in 1932–1934), the reported incidence of episiotomy typically ranged between 40% and 50% for all vaginal deliveries and closer to 80–100% for mothers giving birth for the first time. In the following decades, the use of episiotomy was often reported to be even higher, in many cases exceeding 80% of all vaginal deliveries.

Pleas for the prophylactic and routine use of episiotomy

In the USA and Canada the replacement of emergency episiotomy with routine episiotomy resulted largely from a crusade to encourage the elective use of episiotomy which took place roughly between 1915 and 1935. During this time, episiotomy advocates called for the operation to be performed not as a last resort but prophylactically. As one of these episiotomy protagonists declared:

'Episiotomy should be performed for prophylactic purposes and not as an emergency requirement. It should be a method of choice and not one of necessity' (Deutschman, 1924:CLI).

A closer examination of the drive for prophylactic episiotomy reveals that it occurred in two quite distinct phases. Initially, during the second and third decades of the twentieth century (approximately between 1915 and 1925), a small number of leading obstetrician/gynaecologists made the case for the prophylactic or elective use of episiotomy. During the second phase of the episiotomy crusade (from the mid-1920s through the 1930s), a larger number of somewhat less

Table 3.1 Selected episiotomy rates reported in the literature (1930–1979).

Date	Institution/physician	Overall epis. rate	Primip. rate (when stated)	No. of deliveries	Type of episiotomy % median % mediolateral (when stated)	
1930	Johns Hopkins, Baltimore	0.7		954		
	Chicago Lying-in Hospital	45.1	est. 90–95%	6031		
	5th Avenue Hospital, New York	27.3	est. 90–95%	737		
	Flower Hospital, New York (Tritsch, 1930)	22.3	est. 90–95%	337		
1930	Royal Victoria Hospital, Montreal (Duncan, 1930)	*	vast majority	4025		
1935	Evanston Hospital, Illinois (Galloway, 1935)	*	96%	500		
1 July 1932–30 June 1934	Chicago Lying-in Center (Homebirths) (Buxbaum, 1936)	2.3		*		
1 July 1933–30 June 1935	Chicago Lying-in Hospital (Kretzchmar & Huber, 1938)	52.9	in nearly every instance	5624		
1933–1935	Dr Martin Diethelm	51.0		1587		
	Dr Martin Diethelm (Diethelm, 1938)	50.2		664		
1936–1939	Province of Alberta (Conn et al. 1941)	47.3	77%	2000		
1940	Boston Lying-in Hospital (Nelson & Abramson, 1941)	58.5		2000	40.8	17.1
1935–1946 1938–1946	University Hospital, Baltimore Baltimore City Hospital (Kaltreider & McClelland Dixon, 1948)	37.0		43 503	35	2
June 1948–February 1949	Mercy Hospital, San Diego (Smith, 1951)	54.0		2771	100	

Continued

Table 3.1   Selected episiotomy rates reported in the literature (1930–1979) (*Continued*).

Date	Institution/physician	Overall epis. rate	Primip. rate (when stated)	No. of deliveries	Type of episiotomy % median (when stated)	% mediolateral (when stated)
1 May 1948–30 April 1951	Drs D'Errico and McKeogh (D'Errico & McKeogh, 1951)	89.0	89%	153		
1951	Milwaukee Hospital (Hofmeister, 1952)	86.4		3017	78	8.4
1949–1953	Emanuel Hospital, Portland, Oregon (Fulsher & Fearl, 1955)					
1949		81.0		4233	13.6	62.4
1950		84.0		4293	19.6	64.6
1951		83.0		4493	27.7	55.4
1952		83.0		4837	29.4	53.7
1953		75.0		5393	33.3	41.4
1 January 1952–1 July 1954	Two hospitals, St Petersburg, Florida (Cunningham & Pilkington, 1955)	96.9		290		
1949–1954	Private and Clinical Obstetric Services Dept of OBS University of Washington School of Medicine, Saint Louis (Ballew & Sullivan, 1958)					
1949		59.4		3144		
1950		53.6		3506		
1951		47.6		3751		
1952		38.5		4014		
1953		44.7		4110		
1954		45.3		4290		
1948/9–1958/9	George Washington University Hospital, Washington (Barter *et al.* 1960)					
1948–1949		80.1		2420	50.2	29.9
1954–1955		79.7		3694	69.9	9.8
1955–1956		80.6		3722	73.3	7.3
1956–1957		78.6		3747	73.9	4.7
1957–1958		79.4		3889	74.7	4.7
1958–1959		79.1		3690	75.2	3.9

Period	Source				
1954–1958	Frances Hospital, Waterloo, Iowa (Miller, 1960)				
1954		49.8	900		
1955		49.4	933		
1956		55.2	997		
1957		54.6	1028		
1958		57.4	905		
1960	Milwaukee Maternity Pavillion (Wendt & Wolfgram, 1961)	84.6	500	84.21	0.4
1953–1960	Drs Sieber and Kroon, Mount Carmel Mercy Hospital, Detroit (Sieber & Kroon, 1962)				
1953		85.6	263	75.7	9.9
1954		87.2	299	78.5	8.7
1955		90.0	256	83	7
1956		96.4	277	89.5	6.9
1957		96.6	274	89	7.6
1958		95.6	259	93.4	6.2
1959		95.9	219	94.9	5
1960		100.0	198	93.4	6.6
1960	University of Maryland, School of Medicine, Washington Hospital Center (Dodek, 1963)	67.9	*		
1 May 1961–30 April 1962		94.0	4022	80	14
No date given 'past decade'	Drs O'Leary and O'Leary (O'Leary & O'Leary, 1965)	95.1	4537	100	
31 January 1975–12 February 1976	Evanston Hospital, Illinois (Hughey et al. 1978)	95.0	500 pts using Lamaze method		
		98.0	500 controls		
1976	University of Washington Hospital, Seattle (Shy & Eschenbach, 1979)	69.0			

* Not reported.

distinguished obstetrician/gynaecologists went further by advocating the routine use of the operation.

Prophylactic episiotomy
(approximately 1915–1925)

At a time when most American and British physicians agreed that episiotomy was a rarely needed emergency procedure, a handful of quite prominent obstetrician/gynaecologists began urging the profession to broaden the indications for episiotomy and to employ it in non-emergency situations. They championed episiotomy as a prophylactic for maternal and infant morbidity and infant mortality. Their rationale for prophylactic episiotomy consisted primarily of four claims:

(1)   Episiotomy prevented perineal lacerations and the resulting maternal morbidity associated with this condition;
(2)   Following an episiotomy, when properly repaired, the perineum returned to its prepregnancy state;
(3)   Episiotomy shortened labour thereby preventing infant morbidity and mortality;
(4)   Episiotomy prevented gynaecological problems which might appear many years after the birth (such conditions as cystocele, rectocele and relaxation of the pelvic floor (uterine prolapse)).

One of the most succinct presentations of the reasons for performing episiotomy prophylactically was put this way:

'1 – It saves the woman the debilitating effects of suffering in the first stage and the physical labor of a prolonged second stage.

2 – It undoubtedly preserves the integrity of the pelvic floor and introitus vulvae and forestalls uterine prolapse, rupture of the vesicovaginal septum and the long train of sequelae previously referred to. Virginal conditions are often restored.

3 – It saves the babies' brains from injuries and from immediate and remote effects of prolonged compression. Incision of the soft parts not alone allows us to shorten the second stage, it also relieves the pressure on the brain and will reduce the amount of idiocy, epilepsy, etc.' (DeLee, 1920a:43).

While allegations that episiotomy prevented perineal lacerations, preserved the tonicity of the perineum and saved fetal lives had been made much earlier by the nineteenth century episiotomy enthusiasts, the assertion that the operation prevented future gynaecological problems was unique and central to the argument for the prophylactic use of episiotomy. Despite considerable agreement about the benefits of the prophylactic use of episiotomy, these authorities often disagreed over which type of episiotomy incision to perform. Some favoured making a mediolateral incision while others preferred the median or midline incision.

The launching of the campaign for prophylactic episiotomy can be traced to the 1915 Annual Meeting of the AGS when Brooke Anspach (1915a; 1915b), an Associate in Gynecology at the University of Pennsylvania, declared that 'episiotomy would reduce the physical incapacity following labor' and 'by facilitating delivery would reduce infant mortality and maternal morbidity' (p.714). Three years later before the same Society, Ralph Pomeroy (1918a; 1918b), Associate Professor of Obstetrics and Gynecology at New York's Long Island College Hospital, joined the campaign when he proposed episiotomy for all first-time mothers.

More attention was focused on episiotomy in 1919 when James Harrar (1919a; 1919b; 1919c), Attending Surgeon at the Lying-in Hospital of New York, lobbied obstetricians at the Annual Meeting of the American Association of Obstetricians and Gynecologists (AAOG) to perform elective episiotomy. That same year, Charles Child Jr (1919), Professor of Gynecology at the New York Polyclinic Medical School, presented the proposition of prophylactic episiotomy before the New York City Charity Hospital Alumni Society.

Joseph B. DeLee (1920a; 1920b), Professor of Obstetrics at Northwestern University Medical School, issued the best known plea for prophylactic episiotomy at the 45th Annual Meeting of the AGS in 1920. Two years later, Dan Collier Elkin (1922), an instructor in Obstetrics and Gynecology at Emory University School of Medicine, outlined the prophylactic benefits of episiotomy.

During this period, the last major appeal for the more widespread use of episiotomy was issued in 1924 by David Deutschman (Deutschman, 1924), a New York obstetrician and gynaecologist. For the most part, these prophylactic episiotomy advocates were quite prominent obstetricians/gynaecologists. Anspach, Pomeroy, Harrar and DeLee were Fellows of the American College of Surgeons. Anspach, Pomeroy, DeLee and Child were Fellows of the AGS and Harrar a Fellow of the AAOG. The AAOG, like the AGS, was an elitist specialist society.

The episiotomy crusaders' pleas received substantial attention. Four of them were issued at meetings of the AGS and the AAOG in the presence of many of the most eminent and influential obstetricians in the country. All were widely reported in the medical literature. The papers presented before the AGS and AAOG were included in the published transactions of the meetings (*Transactions of the American Gynecological Society* (Anspach, 1915b; Pomeroy, 1918b; DeLee, 1920b),

Transactions of the American Association of Obstetricians and Gynecologists (Harrar, 1919b), and also published in the *American Journal of Obstetrics and Diseases of Women and Children* (subsequently the *American Journal of Obstetrics and Gynecology*), the official organ of both obstetrical societies (Anspach, 1915a; Pomeroy, 1918a; Harrar, 1919c; DeLee, 1920a). The AGS and AAOG presentations were also abstracted in the *Journal of the American Medical Association*. Two other papers appeared in the *Medical Record* (Child, 1919) and the *Medical Journal and Record* (Deutschman, 1924), both national publications. Elkin's paper (1922), the only one not published in a national journal, appeared in the *Journal of the Medical Association of Georgia*.

Of the physicians campaigning for prophylactic episiotomy, the pleas by Pomeroy and DeLee are most frequently cited by physicians as having influenced obstetrical practice (e.g. Kelly, 1930; Pieri, 1938; Dallas, 1953; Pilkington *et al.*, 1963; Everett & Taylor, 1976; Speert, 1980). Pomeroy, probably best known for devising one of the most popular methods of tubal sterilization (Speert, 1980), generated considerable interest in episiotomy with his 1918 presentation before the AGS provocatively entitled *Shall We Cut and Reconstruct the Perineum for Every Primipara?* (Pomeroy, 1918a).

DeLee, however, was by far the most celebrated and influential physician to champion the prophylactic use of episiotomy. At the time and for decades later, DeLee, a prominent Chicago obstetrician/gynaecologist, exerted substantial influence over the teaching of obstetrics through his widely used textbook *Principles and Practices of Obstetrics* (DeLee, 1913) and his editorship of the *Yearbook of Obstetrics*. In all, DeLee's obstetrical textbook went through 13 editions (1913–1965). He was sole author of the first seven editions and senior author of the next two prior to his death in 1943. DeLee also exerted influence through his position as editor of the *Yearbook of Obstetrics* which he held for nearly four decades (1903–1942).

At the 1920 Annual Meeting of the AGS, DeLee delivered his now famous paper, *The Prophylactic Forceps Operation* (DeLee 1920a;b). In this paper he set out a method for managing normal labour with the purpose of 'relieving pain, supplementing and anticipating the efforts of Nature, reducing the hemorrhage, and preventing and repairing damage' (DeLee, 1920a:34). Prophylactic episiotomy was but one element, albeit a significant one, of the package of obstetric care promoted by DeLee. Essentially, the prophylactic forceps operation consisted of giving morphine and scopolamine (an amnesiac) during the first stage of labour, putting the mother to sleep with ether after the fetal head passed the cervix, performing a mediolateral episiotomy, extracting the infant with forceps, injecting ergot and pituitrin to contract the uterus and prevent postpartum haemorrhage, manually extracting the placenta, repairing the episiotomy incision, and administering more morphine and scopolamine to abolish, as much as possible, the memory of labour.

Many authorities regard DeLee's espousal of the prophylactic forceps and episiotomy as the most enduring of his contributions to obstetrics (Everett & Taylor, 1976; Speert, 1980:187). Furthermore, this paper and what it advocates is regarded by obstetricians and social scientists alike as the cornerstone of modern obstetric practice (Wertz & Wertz, 1979; Shorter, 1990).

Routine episiotomy
(approximately 1925–1935)

Around 1930, a second phase of prophylactic episiotomy activism developed as more rank-and-file obstetrician/gynaecologists began actively lobbying for the universal or indiscriminate use of episiotomy, especially for first-time mothers. It is this universal use of episiotomy that is today, in the minds of most people, synonymous with 'routine' episiotomy.

For the most part, the protagonists of routine episiotomy made all of the same claims about the operation as did the prophylactic episiotomy enthusiasts a decade earlier. However, they, as opposed to their earlier colleagues, explicitly proposed that all, or nearly all, first time mothers would benefit from perineal incision. With the exception of Pomeroy who advised that episiotomy should be performed in every primiparous labour (a practice he later denied doing himself (Pomeroy, 1921)), the other earlier episiotomy enthusiasts never publicly advocated the routine use of the operation.

Also differing from their earlier colleagues, the later advocates of routine episiotomy lacked the stature of a Dr DeLee or Pomeroy. In fact, of the dozen or so advocates of the universal use of episiotomy in the early 1930s, none were Fellows of the AGS, although two were Fellows of the American Association of Obstetricians, Gynecologists and Abdominal Surgeons (Gillis and Hannah). While most of the enthusiasts cannot be counted among the elite of American obstetricians, they were nonetheless specialists in obstetrics and gynaecology. Three were Diplomats of the newly created American Board of Obstetrics and Gynecology (Gillis, Hannah and Galloway) and half were Fellows of the American College of Surgeons (Gillis, Kelly, Hannah, Tritsch and Galloway).

The earlier advocates of prophylactic episiotomy tended to take advantage of national obstetrical meetings to advance their views, but only one later advocate of routine episiotomy lobbied such an audience. Before making its way into print, Gillis' plea (Gillis, 1930) was initially presented as a thesis to the American Association of Obstetricians,

Gynecologists and Abdominal Surgeons in 1929. Many of the appeals for routine episiotomy were, however, made before local professional bodies (Kelly, 1928; 1930; Blevins, 1929; Sellers & Sanders, 1930; Gusman, 1932; Galloway, 1935). Generally speaking about half the pleas appeared in state medical journals such as the *Virginia Medical Monthly* (Kelly, 1928; 1930), the *New Orleans Medical and Surgical Society* (Sellers & Sanders, 1930), the *Ohio Medical Journal* (Gusman, 1932) and the *Illinois Medical Journal* (Galloway, 1935). The remainder were published in more widely distributed national publications such as the *American Journal of Obstetrics and Gynecology* (Blevins, 1929; Hannah, 1930), the *American Journal of Surgery* (Gillis, 1930), *Medical Journal and Record* (Berlind, 1932) and the *Journal of the American Institute of Homeopathy* (Tritsch, 1930).

The role of scientific evidence in prophylactic episiotomy claims-making activities

While many physicians have tended to assume that the success of the pleas for prophylactic episiotomy probably rested on the scientific evidence that showed the operation was safe and beneficial, this was not the case. Although by 1920 there had been significant scientific advances in obstetrics and gynaecology, it is striking that research on episiotomy did not figure prominently in the arguments for its use.

Pomeroy, for example, freely admitted at the time of his talk that there was no evidence for his proposition.

'As sufficient time for labor test will not accrue for another year or two, I can only offer this proposition as a tentative one, lacking entirely present evidence of favorable follow-up results' (Pomeroy, 1918a:219).

As the following passage from Elkin's paper indicates, personal experience with the operation rather than scientific evidence of benefit were the basis of his pleas for prophylactic episiotomy.

'By this procedure, as simple and easy to repair as a first degree laceration, we have restored the vaginal canal to an almost virginal condition, and in no case has vaginal relaxation followed. However, the time elapsing from delivery to follow-up examination has been too short in most cases to make an absolute statement in this regard' (Elkin, 1923:229).

Even the claims made for episiotomy by the eminent Dr DeLee were based entirely upon his personal clinical experience.

'Many efforts are being made to ease the travail of the woman and to better the lot of the infant. What follows is another such effort. Experience alone can decide whether it accomplishes its purpose' (DeLee, 1920a:34).

As Klein (1988) has also pointed out, DeLee's prophylactic forceps operation is particularly notable for the complete absence of references.

At the Annual Meeting of the AGS in 1921, the year following DeLee's dramatic presentation of the prophylactic forceps operation, a discussion erupted over the lack of evidence for the many new obstetrical interventions, including prophylactic use of episiotomy, being proposed and used. At this meeting, Rudolph Holmes, a Chicago obstetrician, generated considerable debate when he accused DeLee, Pomeroy and others of meddlesome midwifery. Holmes pointed out that these physicians:

'... produced no evidence to show that their systems are more worthy, less risky, and promise a higher conservation of life than carefully watched spontaneous labour' (Holmes, 1921:236).

Responding to Holmes' accusations, DeLee admitted there was still little hard evidence supporting his claims about the prophylactic forceps operation made the previous year. Referring to this operation, DeLee admitted to Holmes, 'We must ... prove that this interference in labor brings good results, and that in course of time we will *probably* be able to do' (DeLee, 1921:299). During this same discussion, DeLee also commented, 'Statistics in general are very insecure building stones on which to base judgment' (1921:298). This statement would seem to suggest that DeLee was not at all convinced of the need to scientifically demonstrate that obstetrical interventions were beneficial before introducing them into practice.

Two years later, DeLee had still not provided any data showing that prophylactic forceps and episiotomy were beneficial. As Anspach remarked in 1923:

'When we consider the proposition of DeLee we are impressed, from the beginning, with the fact that here there is actually debatable ground and that we must not, even for a moment, compare the prophylactic use of forceps after episiotomy with either Reed's or Potter's proposals [Reed routinely induced labour at term by means of a tube or bag and Potter routinely shortened the second stage of labour by performing podalic version – delivering the fetus feet first]. Indeed, there is some justification in the advocacy of forceps used prophylactically, and yet, after weighing the matter carefully, even here one must decide that interference in a normal case as a routine measure is unwise and that both the mother and the child will do better if Nature is permitted to take its course. DeLee, at present, furnishes no statistics, so far as we know. His last report gave a gross fetal mortality of 3.6 per cent in 9258 cases, but assuredly these cases were not all treated prophylactically with forceps' (Anspach, 1923:98).

In the years that immediately followed, not only did evidence of the benefit of episiotomy fail to emerge, but also, in at least one case, one of the episiotomy enthusiasts actually reported that the operation appeared to be associated with an increased risk of infection. Buried in a paper on functional dystocia presented at the 1922 meeting of the American Association of Obstetricians, Gynecologists and Abdominal Surgeons, Harrar, who had advocated prophylactic episiotomy in 1919, reported:

'It is a matter of comment in the wards that there is more fever after repair of episiotomy wounds than those of spontaneous laceration' (Harrar, 1923:250).

One of the comments made during the discussion of Harrar's paper is suggestive of the extent to which physicians of the time were not interested in evidence-based medicine, at least as it related to the issue of episiotomy. Despite Harrar's declaration that in his hospital more infections followed episiotomies than spontaneous tears, one discussant simply commented:

'The statement that episiotomy is followed by a higher morbidity than spontaneous tears is a surprise. It certainly does not sound logical to me that a clean-cut wound will give more temperature than a laceration which is spontaneous' (Quigley, 1923:295).

The protagonists of routine episiotomy in the 1930s were equally unconcerned about demonstrating that episiotomy was in fact beneficial. None provided any research evidence to justify their calls for its routine use. As was noted in 1935, 'opinions for and against episiotomy have been formed on the basis of individual experience, but no statistical evidence has been compiled to support the claims of either side' (Nugent, 1935:249). Some of these physicians were so convinced of the benefits that they saw no need to support their claims with evidence. They conceded that the rationales offered, combined with a little experience with the operation, should have been enough to persuade any physician to adopt the practice. Some even went so far as to dismiss the notion of systematically studying the benefits of episiotomy because they felt it was impossible to do so. The following quotation from Tritsch represents this type of thinking.

'It is manifestly very difficult to obtain conclusive figures as to the end results [of episiotomy], for the condition of a perineum and allied subjects is largely a matter of personal opinion and the need for subsequent surgical repair is a matter of degree rather than fact. But we feel in the follow-up of cases taken by and large the end results are definitely better where episiotomy is done in the primiparous women as routine than in cases where it is not' (Tritsch, 1930:333).

Two studies eventually did appear in 1935 which purported to provide evidence supporting the prophylactic use of episiotomy.

However, neither actually revealed that the use of episiotomy during a non-operative delivery (i.e. a spontaneous delivery) was prophylactic. In one case, the report was presented as a study of the effects of delivery with and without episiotomy when, in actuality, it was a study of forceps delivery with and without perineal incision. This semantic difference reveals the extent to which forceps delivery had come to be taken for granted as the usual mode of delivery.

Nevertheless, the study by Nugent of the Philadelphia Lying-in Hospital compared the outcomes of 130 forceps deliveries in which an episiotomy was performed with the outcomes of 72 forceps deliveries in which no perineal incision was performed. Twenty-one per cent of those women who had received an episiotomy during their forceps delivery suffered morbidity (infection) as against 14% who had not. Unable to explain away this finding by differences in the 'complicated operative incidence' between the two groups, Nugent (1935:251) was forced to conclude that 'there is a substantial increase in morbidity attributable to episiotomy'. Nugent drew attention away from this finding by focusing attention on another type of morbidity. Upon examination six weeks postpartum, 45% of the women who had not received an episiotomy showed some failure of restoration of the pelvic floor and perineum (pelvic relaxation, small cystocele, large cystocele) compared with 26% of women who had received an episiotomy. However, in light of all of the results of his study, Nugent was unable to support calls for the routine use of episiotomy.

'Inasmuch as 9.4% of primiparas can be delivered without laceration and without demonstrable anatomic injury at follow up, and inasmuch as an additional 19.8%, though lacerated, show a Grade A result, we are not ready to join Gusman and Tritsch in their campaign for prophylactic episiotomy. We are ready, however, to paraphrase the old surgical dictum and say, "When in doubt, cut"' (Nugent, 1935:255).

In contrast to Nugent who compared the end-results of forceps deliveries with and without episiotomy, a second study compared spontaneous labour without episiotomy to labours in which prophylactic forceps and episiotomy were used. This study, conducted at the Woman's Hospital of New York City by Aldridge and Watson, compared 2800 primipara delivered on their ward between 1920–1925 and 1930–1934. These two time periods were used because spontaneous deliveries were more common during the 1920–1925 period and prophylactic methods of delivery during the 1930–1934 period. Completely ignoring the issue of whether or not performing an episiotomy during spontaneous labour was beneficial, Aldridge and Watson focused instead on forceps deliveries performed with and without episiotomy. They concluded:

'Perineal incision when used in conjunction with any type of vaginal operation delivery consistently reduced the incidence of birth injuries and postpartum complications' (Aldridge & Watson, 1935:565).

The absence of strong evidence showing that routine episiotomy was indeed prophylactic as claimed continued into the 1940s. A 1942 report on a study of post-partum pelvic tissue damage of 1000 women ended by stating:

'Conclusions regarding the controversial subject of routine episiotomy were avoided at this time because of an insufficient number of cases. Suffice it to say that both those with and without episiotomy suffered damage. Protagonists of either procedure need more detailed and objective evidence in order that unified thought and practice may benefit the parturient woman' (Gainey, 1943).

Quite clearly, the advocacy of prophylactic and routine episiotomy during the 1920s and 1930s was not based on any evidence that the operation was beneficial. By extension, the subsequent adoption of routine episiotomy by American physicians was equally not influenced by scientific research or reasoning. What then explains the rather sudden increase in popularity of episiotomy?

Factors encouraging physicians to adopt routine episiotomy

While research may have had little to do with the overwhelming acceptance the operation received between the mid-teens and 1930s, a number of other factors greatly facilitated its widespread use. In large part, changes that were simultaneously occurring in the ideology and practice of obstetrics encouraged physicians to resort to the operation frequently.

The 'childbirth as pathology' argument

One of the most important reasons for the acceptance of routine episiotomy had to do with a shift in the conceptualization of the nature of childbirth which was taking place in obstetrics during the 1920s and 1930s. As described in Chapter 2, a major impediment to the success of the nineteenth century episiotomy enthusiasts was the incompatibility between surgical intervention and the existing belief system in obstetrics. These early beliefs held that childbirth and the functioning of the perineum were normal or physiological processes. The prophylactic episiotomy protagonists of the early twentieth century attempted to overcome this barrier to the wider use of episiotomy by recasting childbirth as a pathological and pathogenic process. They argued that childbirth was more often than not a faulty and destructive process requiring considerable obstetrical intervention to prevent, minimize and repair the damage incurred during labour and delivery.

The following passages are classical examples of how prophylactic episiotomy enthusiasts argued that childbirth was a pathological process, an argument upon which their entire 'prophylactic' rationale for episiotomy rested. Note the skill with which each makes use of quite dramatic metaphors to argue that normal birth was virtually non-existent.

> 'Every primipara incurs a permanent modification of the pelvic floor in the course of delivery of her full-term child. In a disputed but high percentage of first births the acute stage of this modification presents some extent of open lacerated wound and in nearly all the rest, concealed damage to fascia and levator ani muscles is acknowledged to occur and to be the factor paramount in various degrees of subsequent prolapsus uteri, cystocele and rectocele.' (Pomeroy, 1918a:211).

> '... A long second stage has destroyed innumerable children by prolonged pressure effects and varying degrees of asphyxia. Why should we consider it other than reckless to allow the child's head to be used as a battering ram wherewith to shatter a resisting outlet? Why not open the gates and close them after the procession has passed?' (Pomeroy, 1918a:213).

DeLee presents the 'childbirth as pathology' argument in extremely graphic terms.

> 'Labor has been called, and is still believed by many to be, a normal function. It always strikes physicians as well as laymen as bizarre, to call labor an abnormal function, a disease, and yet it is a decidedly pathologic process. Everything, of course, depends on what we define as normal. If a woman falls on a pitchfork, and drives it through her perineum, we call that pathologic-abnormal, but if a large baby is driven through the pelvic floor, we say that it is natural, and therefore normal. If a baby were to have its head caught in a door very lightly, but enough to cause cerebral hemorrhage, we would say that it is decidedly pathologic, but when a baby's head is crushed against a tight pelvic floor, and a hemorrhage in the brain kills it, we call this normal, at least we say that the function is natural, not pathogenic.
>
> In both cases, the cause of the damage, the fall on the pitchfork, and the crushing of the door, is pathogenic, that is disease producing, and in the same sense labor is pathogenic, disease producing, and anything pathogenic is pathologic or abnormal.
>
> Now you will say that the function of labor is normal, that only those cases which result in disease may be called abnormal. Granted, but how many labor cases, measured by modern standards, may be so classified? ... it amounts to the majority today. In fact, only a small minority of women escape damage during labor, while 4 per cent of the babies are killed and a

large indeterminable number are more or less injured by the direct action of the natural process itself. So frequent are these bad effects, that I have often wondered whether Nature did not deliberately intend women should be used up in the process of reproduction, in a manner analogous to that of the salmon, which dies after spawning? Perhaps laceration, prolapse and all the evils soon to be mentioned are, in fact, natural to labor and therefore normal, in the same way as the death of the mother salmon and the death of the male bee in copulation, are natural and normal. If you adopt this view, I have no ground to stand on, but, if you believe that a woman after delivery should be as healthy, as well, as anatomically perfect as she was before, and that the child should be undamaged, then you will have to agree with me that labor is pathogenic, because experience has proved such ideal results exceedingly rare' (DeLee, 1920a:39–41).

Overcoming initial resistance to prophylactic episiotomy

That the episiotomy protagonists' claims-making activities were indeed challenging the existing belief system in obstetrics is evident in the criticisms initially attracted by their campaigning. When they first advanced the notion of prophylactic episiotomy, the episiotomy advocates encountered considerable resistance from some fairly prominent physicians who continued to believe birth was a normal process not requiring prophylactic surgical intervention. Although the comments made by the discussants attending Pomeroy's talk before the AGS suggest his paper was positively received, other notable physicians were not impressed.

John Whitridge Williams, considered 'the Dean of Obstetricians' at the time, rejected Pomeroy's proposition and continued advocating the accepted obstetric formula of delivering all women with as little interference as possible (Dallas, 1953). Williams was Professor of Obstetrics at Johns Hopkins University, Dean of the medical school, Obstetrician-in-Chief to the Johns Hopkins Hospital, and an ex-president of the AGS (1914). He was also the author of a widely used textbook *Obstetrics: A Text-book for the Use of Students and Practitioners* (following Williams' death it was eventually renamed *Williams Obstetrics*). From the first edition of his textbook in 1906, Williams had little use for episiotomy. He acknowledged that many authorities advised performing an episiotomy when a rupture of the perineum seemed imminent, but he did not accept the claim that episiotomy prevented perineal lacerations or healed better than a spontaneous laceration.

'Personally, I see no advantage in the procedure, as my experience is that ordinarily perineal tears will heal almost uniformly if properly sutured and cared for' (Williams, 1906:289).

In the fifth edition of his textbook in 1926, the edition following Pomeroy's plea for prophylactic episiotomy, Williams inserted another paragraph denouncing the practice. While not challenging the claim that episiotomy might be a prophylaxis for postpartum gynaecological problems, he maintained his disapproval of elective perineal incision.

'In an article entitled "Shall we cut and reconstruct the perineum for every primipara?", Pomeroy, in 1918, advocated making a midline incision as soon as the perineum begins to bulge, with the idea that its accurate repair immediately after delivery would prevent the development of relaxation of the pelvic floor in the future. While this may be so, it would appear to be an inadvisable routine procedure for two reasons: first, that it converts every labor into an operative one, and second, that if ideally successful its repetition would be logically called for at each subsequent delivery' (Williams, 1926:357).

As for DeLee, he too was strongly criticized when he first advanced prophylactic episiotomy and forceps. Many denounced the operation as radical. Following the presentation of his paper before the AGS in 1920, there were few positive comments concerning his talk. By and large, the discussants were not convinced that childbirth was almost always pathological as DeLee claimed and were therefore quite hesitant to accept the position that surgical intervention in childbirth was really necessary let alone prophylactic. As the first discussant, Williams set the tone for the discussion by emphatically disagreeing with DeLee.

'I am sorry to say that there are only two things in Dr DeLee's paper with which I entirely agree. The first is to allow the cervix to undergo spontaneous dilatation, and the second is the correctness of the general anatomical considerations which he has adduced. With the rest I do not agree. Doubtless Dr DeLee, or the majority of those present, can deliver women in the manner he has described and leave them in better condition than had they been delivered in the usual way by the average practitioner. On the other hand, I believe that if his practice were to become general and widely adopted, women would be worse off, eventually than had their labors been conducted by midwives' (Williams, 1920:77).

Williams concluded his comments by stating:

'If I have understood Dr DeLee correctly, it seems to me that he interferes 19 times too often out of 20. Of course what I say applies to normal labors. . . . I therefore believe should his recommendation be generally adopted that it would do an immense amount of harm and far counterbalance the good which it may accomplish in his expert hands' (Williams, 1920:77).

Other discussants such as Thomas Watts Eden, a distinguished English obstetrician and invited guest, and American obstetricians

Henry Byford of Chicago and Edward Davis of Philadelphia vocalized the then widely accepted view of childbirth as a physiological process usually not requiring surgical intervention. As Byford put it:

> 'I think the whole gist of the subject is that of Dr DeLee recommending this procedure in all cases. . . . The fact that so many cases get well of themselves where they are left to Nature shows that the procedure should be used in the individual case, not as a routine method' (Byford, 1920:79).

Within a decade, the obstetrical belief system had changed in the direction Pomeroy and DeLee had advocated. Childbirth had been successfully recast as a pathological process. As the following passage from one of the routine episiotomy protagonists reveals, the pathogenic nature of 'normal' labour was no longer debatable but had become widely accepted.

> 'That the tissues of the modern woman do not well withstand the tension and stretching incident to the average normal labor and that injuries to the pelvic soft parts occur in the great majority of so-called normal labors is a *well-known fact*' (Gillis, 1930:520,522).

So strongly had the conceptualization of childbirth as a pathological process taken hold in obstetrics that by the time routine episiotomy was being advocated in the 1930s, opposition to prophylactic episiotomy had virtually completely dissipated. Even Williams, the most influential opponent of the operation, had softened his position. In the sixth edition of his textbook, the last one authored by Williams himself, he replaced the judgemental sentence stating he saw 'no advantage in the procedure' with the more neutral 'I rarely employ the operation'. For the first time he also recognized that the operation had supporters and was used often.

> 'On the other hand, many of my associates resort to it frequently, so that it may be said that its employment is largely a matter of taste' (Williams, 1930:282).

Clearly, the success episiotomy enthusiasts had in encouraging the prophylactic use of episiotomy was inextricably linked to eventual acceptance by the obstetrical profession of childbirth as a pathological process. Without this change in the obstetrical belief system, opposition to the prophylactic routine use of episiotomy likely would have continued. Furthermore, once childbirth was recast in pathological terms, the obstetrical profession naturally placed renewed emphasis on prevention of the damage believed to be caused by childbirth. As one obstetrician of the time put it:

'To discharge the patient at the end of the puerperium as well as she was before she became pregnant is the supreme test of the competent obstetric practice and the only one by which our work should be judged. This well-being or fitness applies as well to the integrity of the perineum and the pelvic floor, the size of the vagina and the proper supports of the pelvic organs as to the general constitutional health of the mother and child' (Gillis, 1930:523).

Changes in obstetrical practice

Changes in obstetrical practice also had a strong effect on physicians' episiotomy use. As several obstetricians have pointed out over the years, episiotomy became a significant part of obstetrical care only with the shift of obstetrics from home to hospital (Parks & Barter, 1954; Barter *et al.*, 1960). This shift took place during the first part of the twentieth century. Wertz and Wertz (1979:135) estimate that between 1900 and 1940, hospital births increased from less than 5% to 50% of all births. In urban areas particularly, hospital deliveries increased dramatically during the 1920s, and by 1939 75% of all urban women were having their babies in hospitals.

The moving of childbirth into hospital directly affected the use of episiotomy in at least two ways.

(1)   It facilitated the use of the operation by making the technology necessary to safely carry out the procedure readily available to obstetricians. Physicians attending hospital deliveries were encouraged to use episiotomy more frequently because many of the practical impediments they encountered at homebirths were not present at hospital births. As one obstetrician remarked:

> 'Without anesthesia, proper lighting, capable assistants, adequate exposure, and the availability of aseptic technique in the home, incisions and lacerations of the perineum were avoided whenever possible' (Barter *at al.*, 1960:655).

(2)   The phenomenon known as the 'cascade of intervention' refers to the situation whereby one particular obstetrical intervention necessitates or encourages further intervention(s) to counteract the effects of the initial action (MacLennan, 1978; Inch, 1984). Applying this concept, as more women delivered in hospital and as increasing numbers of them received both obstetrical anaesthesia and forceps (separately and combined), the use of episiotomy increased correspondingly. Anaesthesia, by interfering with the natural expulsion efforts of the mother, increased the need for forceps which in turn encouraged the use of episiotomy as perineal incision provides greater room for the application of

forceps. In the same vein, both general anaesthesia and forceps were associated with the increasing use of lithotomy position which also increases the chances of the need for episiotomy. As Wertz and Wertz point out:

> '...one technique could often require the use of another. Anesthesia was counteracted by oxytocin; episiotomy required local anesthesia; forceps required anesthesia and episiotomy; the lithotomy position required episiotomy' (1979:165).

While there are no national statistics documenting the increasing use of anaesthesia, forceps, lithotomy position or episiotomy during the 1920s and 1930s, there is evidence this is what occurred. As one obstetrician in the early 1950s noted:

> '...The introduction of Nebutal into obstetric practice and the rapid improvement of anesthetic technics further increased the use of outlet forceps with episiotomy' (Dallas, 1953:29).

See also Aldridge and Watson's (1935) historical cohort study of episiotomy (pages 45–6). Between 1925 and 1930, the prophylactic forceps operation became common practice at this hospital with a resulting increase in the use of episiotomy as well.

Physician convenience and the desire to control the uncertainty of childbirth

The greater use of episiotomy during the 1930s can also be traced to its promotion as a means of making the birth process more predictable and thereby facilitating the work of obstetricians. As the historian Leavitt has noted, this was a time when 'hospital-based obstetricians did develop routines for managing childbirth that incorporated systematic use of pain-relieving drugs, labor inducers and technological intervention' (1983:298).

While all of the 1930s advocates of routine episiotomy reiterated with great conviction the claims about the alleged benefits of prophylactic episiotomy made by DeLee and his colleagues, some also reintroduced the late nineteenth-century rationale that episiotomy was a convenient means of reducing the unpredictability of perineal lacerations. By performing an episiotomy, they claimed that the physician, not nature, determined the location and extent of the perineal wound. It also meant that by performing an episiotomy the physician no longer had to anticipate the possible occurrence of a perineal laceration. The episiotomy, done at the physician's discretion, replaced the unpredictable, and therefore uncontrollable, laceration.

'The substitution of episiotomy for laceration is but replacing a jagged and irregular wound by a clean regular incision, placed to the surgeon's judgment and better adapted to surgical repair' (Danforth, 1928:508).

'We are definitely cognizant of the fact that a straight incised wound in a preconceived location is much safer and heals better than a ragged wound which may choose some dangerous route for extension' (Lubin, 1932:81).

As the above passages also imply, many of the routine episiotomy advocates of the 1930s also reintroduced the notion that episiotomies were easier to repair than a spontaneous laceration. They alleged that because episiotomy incisions were straight surgical incisions they required less skill to repair than a spontaneous 'jagged' or 'irregular' laceration. This meant episiotomies were both easier and quicker to suture.

'When we consider this fact [the frequency of perineal tears] we can fully appreciate the greater wisdom of incision which is sharp and clean and allows for approximation in suturing, to a tear which is very often ragged and difficult of approximation' (Tritsch, 1930:329).

'Episiotomy substitutes a clean straight incision for a jagged irregular lacerated wound. The more extensive laceration may be so long, so jagged, or so undermining that its repair may constitute a very difficult task' (Cooke, 1937:413).

In the context of the general acceptance of the pathological nature of childbirth and the rapidly rising number of hospital births during the 1930s, performing episiotomy for physician convenience may have been a compelling reason for increasingly overworked obstetricians to opt for the operation. Physicians working in hospital often found themselves caring for several women in the second stage of labour at the same time. By performing the procedure, they no longer had to worry about the possibility of a laceration and all the sequelae associated with this negative outcome. As one obstetrician remarked in the 1920s:

'Any procedure which tends to lessen irksomeness and burdens will find a ready ear in the profession' (Schumman in Applegate, 1924).

Physicians also believed episiotomy shortened labour allowing them to more quickly complete a birth so that they could get on to the next patient; it was a means of streamlining the childbirth assembly line.

Additional evidence that physician convenience played some role in episiotomy's increasing popularity comes from the writings of physicians belonging to the conservative school of obstetric thought. These physicians, who were otherwise opposed to elective obstetrical intervention, preferred the practice of 'watchful expectancy' – waiting until intervention proved necessary. Even among such conservatively minded physicians, however, episiotomy was still strongly embraced. For example, William C. Danforth, Attending Gynecologist and Obstetrician at Evanston Hospital, Illinois was a believer in conservative obstetrics, but was nevertheless 'strongly in favor of episiotomy in primipara' when lacerations appeared likely (1922:611). He also believed repaired incisions healed better than lacerations.

The transformation of obstetrics and gynaecology during the 1920s and 1930s

In obstetrics, the period roughly between 1920 and 1940 can be characterized as a period of professional 'transformation'. Bucher describes the process of occupational transformation in the following way:

'Basically, there is fundamental redefinition of the nature of the field, of the underlying paradigm, of the territory, of the mission, of all of these. In carrying out this sort of redefinition, the transforming field must undergo equally fundamental alterations in its relationship with formal organizations, other occupations, or client groups. It must repudiate older images and set forth new rhetoric to justify and clarify the new roles it wishes to establish in organizations' (1988:145).

Summey and Hurst's analysis of the obstetrical literature between the 1920s and 1940s describes these years in the history of the obstetrical profession as 'a period of professional establishment, characterized by self-definition, boundary setting and defensiveness of its past performance' (1986:136). It was at this time that the formal alliance between obstetrics and gynaecology developed in the USA. Most importantly, the period marks the emergence of interventionist obstetrics as the new dominant belief system influencing obstetrical and gynaecological practice (Wertz & Wertz, 1979; Summey & Hurst, 1986).

The development of this new professional identity can be traced to the 45th Annual Meeting of the AGS in 1920. In his Presidential Address, Robert Dickinson declared, 'the point is come where old fields must give new crops and new lands be opened up or our claims surrendered' (1920:1). He presented a four-year plan to professionalize the field and delineate its role in medicine. The elements of his plan consisted of:

- the need to develop a standard nomenclature of diseases and operations (i.e. develop a common vocabulary);
- establish certain standards in obstetrics and gynaecology;

- improve teaching;
- increase involvement in social issues related to reproduction;
- certify specialists;
- train more leaders;
- increase the number of women in the field; and
- establish a journal.

Dickinson's address was followed by DeLee's paper on prophylactic forceps and the pathogenic nature of labour, which laid the foundation for the future of active obstetric intervention in childbirth. Symbolic of the new direction the profession was embarking on, the first volume of the newly founded *American Journal of Obstetrics and Gynecology* opened with Dickinson's Presidential Address and included DeLee's prophylactic forceps paper.

In their paper, Summey and Hurst (1986) trace the transformation of the obstetrical profession through the debates which erupted over activist ideology. The following passage illustrates this debate.

'Just now, obstetrics is upset by a strong radical school, which is attempting to change its point of view from physiology to surgery' (Lynch, 1924:398).

As the passage above implies, the so-called 'radicals' argued in favour of interventionist obstetrics (operative intervention along the lines proposed by DeLee) while the so-called 'conservatives' preferred the concept of watchful expectancy (waiting until intervention proved necessary). Paradoxically, Anspach who had himself advocated the greater use of episiotomy in 1915, a few years later disparagingly describes the new obstetrics sweeping the profession. This passage describes the context in which the advocacy of routine episiotomy was taking place during the early 1920s.

'At the present day, Nature no longer dominates the practice of obstetrics. The modern obstetrician no longer patiently awaits her pleasure, assisting only when it becomes evident that help is necessary. Today, on the slightest provocation and often on decidedly uncertain grounds, he takes matters into his own hands. He is not content even to await the onset of labor but takes steps to induce it at the time when he believes the process should occur. After the cervix has become dilated, or when it is easily dilatable, he turns the child *in utero* and delivers it feet first, or if the head of the child has reached the perineal floor, he completes delivery at once by means of episiotomy and the aid of forceps. If a case promises to be difficult, he ignores the natural channel of expulsion and delivers the child through an abdominal incision' (Anspach, 1923:96).

Prophylactic episiotomy, and the initial resistance to it which I have already described, was in many cases one element of this larger debate about the state of obstetrics and where it should be going. Where DeLee and the other radicals argued that childbirth was, and should be, seen as pathogenic, the conservatives opposed this conceptualization of labour by retaining the view of childbirth as an essentially normal process that should be treated as such.

'The basic error has crept into the obstetric field that pregnancy and labor are pathologic entities, that childbearing is a disease, a surgical malady which must be terminated by some spectacular procedure. There is too insistent preachment by those who are defining a reign of terror, of promiscuous operative furor, by the argument that women have so degenerated that childbearing is a phase of pathologic anatomy' (Holmes, 1921:233).

Furthermore, the 'childbirth as pathology' argument which underpins the radical school of obstetrical thought also served to justify the use of episiotomy on the basis of the alleged prophylactic benefits of the operation. Not surprisingly, all prophylactic interventions proposed to prevent or minimize childbirth pathology, which was thought always to occur, were rapidly taken up by obstetricians. At the same time, prophylactic episiotomy, like the prophylactic forceps operation, was symbolic of the new interventionist ideology as well as representing the conscious rejection of the age-old belief that birth was normal. Performing prophylactic episiotomy, therefore, was a simple way for an obstetrician to acknowledge that he was an adherent of the new surgical obstetrics.

On a more practical level, prophylactic episiotomy played into the hands of some obstetrician's preoccupation with status by distinguishing them from midwives and generalists. As Summey and Hurst note, 'external pressure for better education and training of obstetricians, and internal pressure to raise the status of the profession, resulted in a move to close ranks' (1986:142). One example of this was the establishment of the American Board of Obstetrics and Gynecology (ABOG) in 1930 to certify specialists in the field. One of the rationales behind the formation of the ABOG was that certification would help elevate the standards and advance the cause of obstetrics and gynaecology by raising the status of the profession (Dannreuther, 1931). In establishing the ABOG, the obstetrical 'specialists' were suggesting that their methods had more to offer than those of the midwives or generalists. As the following quotations from two of the routine episiotomy protagonists indicate, episiotomy was touted as one of those methods.

'The question is often raised "should we make so many of our deliveries surgical procedures?" If we are to elevate the obstetrics above the old-fashioned midwifery and if our ultimate goal is to discharge our patient with her birth canal as nearly to its pre-pregnancy state as possible, then we

certainly cannot afford to be timid about such a simple procedure as episiotomy. The answer is obvious' (Gusman, 1932:653).

'First, we do not recommend the operation of episiotomy routinely in home
confinements excepting under the most ideal conditions. Secondly, we do
not recommend routine episiotomy by those untrained in obstetric surgery.
In conclusion ... the operation should only be performed under ideal hospital conditions by one qualified in obstetric surgery' (Tritsch, 1930:333).

At the same time that episiotomy served to distance obstetrics from
'old-fashioned midwifery', the operation also appealed to obstetricians
with surgical aspirations. By performing episiotomy, obstetricians
could feel they were using their surgical skills which were more greatly
valued than their 'midwifery' skills. Another indication of the
increasing interest of obstetricians to be associated with surgical skills
was the renaming in 1920 of the American Association of Obstetricians
and Gynecologists to the American Association of Obstetricians,
Gynecologists and Abdominal Surgeons. Davis-Floyd, an anthro-
pologist, offers the following complementary interpretation of the
motivation of obstetricians to align themselves with surgery.

'The episiotomy is also conceptually useful to obstetrics. From its inception,
the obstetrical profession was constrained to justify itself as being equal to
other branches of medicine in which the inherent pathology of the disease or
accident being treated was perhaps clearer than is the inherent "pathology"
of natural childbirth. Since surgery constitutes the central core of Western
medicine, the ultimate form of manipulation of the human body-machine,
the legitimation of obstetrics necessitated the transformation of childbirth
into a surgical procedure. Routinizing the episiotomy has proven to be an
effective means of accomplishing this transformation' (Davis-Floyd,
1988:168).

Simply put, routine episiotomy was an integral part of the overwhelming acceptance of interventionist obstetrics and the pathological
nature of childbirth which took place in the 1930s. As Arthur Bill, a
quite distinguished obstetrician and gynaecologist, announced in his
Presidential Address to the American Association of Obstetricians,
Gynecologists and Abdominal Surgeons in 1931, 'the new school of
obstetrics ... is without doubt here to stay' (Bill, 1932:162). From this
perspective, the routinization of episiotomy is illustrative of the
transformation of obstetrics which took the form of the 'new obstetrics'
with its ideology of intervention.

Before concluding this chapter, I would like to present one other
explanation for the acceptance of routine episiotomy which has been
suggested in the literature. This alternative theory, however, is not
supported by the data presented above.

'Discovery of the fetus'

Edward Shorter, a medical historian at the University of Toronto, has advanced the thesis that the 'discovery of the fetus' in the 1930s caused a substantial increase in obstetrical intervention, including the routinization of episiotomy. He argues that before 1930 little medical attention had been given to the condition of the infant at birth. All obstetric interventions he contends were directed toward sparing the mother. This all changed in the 1930s, he claims, because doctors began considering the infant's condition as a reason for intervening in the labour. As Shorter (1990) puts it:

'Toward 1930 the fetus was "discovered". One cannot date this *prise de conscience* exactly, but certainly in the late 1920s and early 1930s there was a trend toward sparing the infant in delivery. Particularly in America "fetal indications" began to be accepted for obstetric operations, in addition to "maternal indications". In plain language, this means intervening in birth to help the child even if the mother is perfectly all right' (p. 166).

Specifically regarding episiotomy, Shorter argues that prior to 1930 the operation was strictly used because it was easier to repair than a spontaneous perineal laceration. After 1930 he suggests episiotomies were done primarily for the sake of the infant.

'But only in the 1930s did the infant start to figure in the reasons for doing an episiotomy. As a result, the frequency of the operation increased significantly. The new logic was to spare the child a prolonged expulsive stage of labor. Enlarging the vaginal outlet would permit speedy forceps delivery of its head. When in 1937 an obstetrical surgeon justified the high frequency of episiotomies, he placed "fetal indications" first: "the fetus is protected from the effects of a prolonged second stage, particularly from certain injuries which may result when the head acts as a dilator of the mother's soft parts" ... Joseph DeLee's textbook mentions protecting the fetus for the first time in 1933. *Williams Obstetrics'* first reference appeared in 1950: "spares the baby's head the necessity of serving as a battering ram"' (Shorter, 1990:172).

While I do not dispute that, in general, the fetus became a new focal point in obstetrics during the 1930s, this did not produce the routine-use episiotomy as Shorter claims. Shorter's interpretation of what brought about routine episiotomy in the 1930s is inaccurate. The 'evidence' he presents to support his thesis is selective and misleading.

In the first place, the rationale that episiotomy can save the life of the fetus was well known and accepted before the 1930s. Both Ould in 1742 (Parvin, 1882) and Stahl in 1895 promoted episiotomy as a means of saving the life of an infant. The following quotation is from a paper presented at the 1904 Annual Meeting of the AGS by J. Clifton Edgar, a prominent New York obstetrician and author of one of the major American obstetrics texts of the early twentieth century. As the passage indicates, as early as the turn of the century many obstetricians considered saving the infant a priority over saving the perineum.

'Preservation of the structures of the pelvic floor during the passage of the fetal head and shoulders has been placed by some authorities as second in importance only to preservation of the lives of the mother and child' (Edgar, 1904:208).

Furthermore, during the second and third decades of the twentieth century, the rationale that episiotomy prevented or reduced infant mortality and morbidity received considerable attention from many influential protagonists of prophylactic episiotomy (Anspach, 1915a; Pomeroy, 1918a; Child, 1919; Harrar, 1919b; DeLee, 1920a;b).

Secondly, Shorter's suggestion that during the 1930s fetal indications for episiotomy replaced maternal indications as the primary reason for undertaking the operation is simply not true. Some physicians of the 1930s championed routine episiotomy on the grounds that it prevented infant morbidity and mortality (namely cerebral haemorrhage and death in premature babies) (e.g. Berlind, 1932). However, many more episiotomy enthusiasts advocated the universal use of the operation because they believed it was a prophylactic for maternal trauma, specifically postpartum gynaecological problems and perineal lacerations (e.g. Blevins, 1929; Gillis, 1930; Hannah, 1930; Kelly, 1930; Sellers & Sanders, 1930; Tritsch, 1930; Gusman, 1932; Galloway, 1935).

The quotation by the 'obstetrical surgeon' Shorter presents is deceptive. Shorter fails to note that the paper that immediately followed the one by the 'obstetrical surgeon' is devoted entirely to the issue of the management of maternal birth injuries. In the second paper by another prominent obstetrician (Cooke, 1937), episiotomy is touted exclusively as a prophylaxis against laceration of the perineum. In that article, fetal indications for performing the operation are not even mentioned. When both these articles are considered together, it is not at all clear that a shift in the prioritization of the indications for episiotomy had taken place as Shorter implies.

Concerning Shorter's reference to DeLee, it should be remembered that at least 13 years earlier, DeLee in his 1920 paper expounded upon the dangers of labour to the infant and offered episiotomy as a means of saving babies' 'brains from injuries' (DeLee, 1920a:43). Shorter's reference to *Williams Obstetrics* is also misleading in that he is suggesting this textbook 'discovered' the fetus as a reason for performing the operation in 1950. He neglects to say that this is also the first edition of *Williams Obstetrics* to unequivocally endorse routine episiotomy for any reason; maternal or fetal. As described above, in the first six

editions of the text written by Williams himself, he advised that episiotomy was not necessary and discredited the common maternal
indications suggested for performing the operation. He was unconvinced of the claims that episiotomies were easier to repair and healed
better than a spontaneous perineal tear.

Shorter's theory does not appear to be supported by the data.
Therefore the 'discovery of the fetus' is an unlikely explanation for the
introduction of routine episiotomy.

Chapter 4

Emergence of the Liberal Use of Episiotomy in the UK

Whereas the routine use of episiotomy had become widely accepted in the USA by the 1940s, the liberal use of episiotomy, as it is sometimes referred to in the UK (Sleep *et al.*, 1984), did not occur until the late 1960s. As illustrated in Fig. 3, the national episiotomy rate for England and Wales began to increase dramatically only between the late 1960s and 1970s. While never quite reaching the heights found in the USA, the episiotomy rate in England more than doubled in 11 years, climbing from 25% of all hospital deliveries in 1967 to 53.4% in 1978 (Macfarlane & Mugford, 1984:245). The sharpest increase occurred during the early 1970s. In some hospitals, the operation was so frequently performed that nearly every first-time mother received an episiotomy (Oakley, 1979; Buchan & Nicholls, 1980; Kitzinger, 1981)

This chapter investigates the reasons for the persistence of restrictive use of episiotomy and then the revision of this practice in favour of its more liberal use. It also shows the importance of identifying the parties interested in adopting an innovation and explaining their use of it. In this case, differentiating between medical and midwifery use of episiotomy led to the identification of different factors that stimulated the use of the operation in each profession.

The restrictive use of episiotomy

During the 1930s in the USA medical consensus favouring the emergency use of episiotomy began to give way to the elective use of episiotomy. In the UK this change did not occur for another three decades. Until the 1960s, physicians continued to view episiotomy as largely an emergency procedure which was seldom necessary in normal deliveries. Reluctance of the medical establishment to adopt elective episiotomy was largely related to the organization of maternity care in the UK. Of primary importance was the distinction between midwifery and obstetrical care and the particular view about the nature of childbirth held by each of these types of care givers.

Obstetrical vs. midwifery care

Where American physicians had succeeded in redefining what had been considered a normal physiological process as a potentially abnormal or pathological one by the 1920s and 1930s, the boundary between 'normal' and 'abnormal' births continues to remain distinct in the UK. In 1902, the Midwives Act was passed by the UK parliament granting midwives the status of independent practitioners. This legislation gave midwives responsibility for 'normal' births. As Oakley (1986) and others (e.g. Anisef & Basson, 1979; Arney, 1985) have observed, the Act legitimized and solidified a division within childbearing between the normal and the abnormal, with midwives becoming 'practitioners in the art of the normal and obstetricians in that of the abnormal' (Oakley, 1986:142).

A further division between midwifery and obstetrical care resulting from this dichotomous view of childbirth concerned the place of birth. Until the 1950s, most women with uncomplicated pregnancies and childbirth were delivered by midwives in their own homes, while obstetricians cared for the abnormal or complicated pregnancies and deliveries in hospital. Over time, the division between midwifery and obstetrical care of childbearing has been quite consistent. Midwives have historically attended and continue to attend the vast majority of deliveries in the UK. In 1946, 90% of deliveries in England and Wales were attended by a midwife, who took full responsibility in over 75% of cases (Oakley, 1986). By the early 1980s, the midwife was still the senior person present in 75% of all deliveries (Task Force on the Implementation of Midwifery in Ontario, 1987:60).

No room for elective episiotomy in normal birth

As long as childbirth was considered a physiological process with domiciliary midwives and general practitioners caring for normal births, British physicians were prepared to endorse the use of episiotomy only as an emergency measure. On a theoretical level, they, like the nineteenth century physicians before them, saw no justification in complicating what they considered a natural process by elective surgical intervention. On a more practical level, British physicians also feared that the adoption of episiotomy would lead to the hospitalization of normal childbirth. Like all operations, they believed that episiotomy should take place in a hospital environment. The influential Scottish physician J.W. Ballentyne expressed these views in 1919 when he denounced the American obstetrician/gynaecologist Pomeroy's plea in 1918 for the widespread use of episiotomy. Disagreeing with

Pomeroy's depiction of childbirth as a pathological process, Ballentyne rhetorically asks:

'Are we really to divide the whole recto-vaginal septum in order to prevent it tearing in part? One is ready to admit the propriety of some such surgical procedure in desperate cases; but then one remembers Pomeroy's inter-rogative paper-title – "for every primipara". One sympathises with the surgical ambition felt by many to make as neat a job of labour as of say, an appendectomy; but dilatation of the sphincter followed by complete incision of the perineum and possibly also of the sphincter challenges inquiry and raises the question whether the perineum can be best protected by tem-porarily abolishing it, and that, as Mr Pepys might have said, "seems pretty strange"' (Ballantyne, 1919:411).

He went on to say that the routine use of episiotomy would turn the first confinement into a 'distinct surgical proposition ... [where] the operating-room should be its environment' (Ballentyne, 1919:411). The following year, Thomas Watts Eden, a prominent consulting obstetric physician at Charing Cross Hospital in London, author of the text *A Manual of Midwifery* (Eden, 1911) and Honorary Fellow of the AGS, rejected the prophylactic use of forceps and episiotomy for the same reasons (Eden, 1920). As is implied by the following passage, the British continued to consider normal childbirth as a physiological as opposed to pathological process leaving little room for elective peri-neal incision. The passage comes from Eden's response to DeLee's 1920 talk on the *The Prophylactic Forceps Operation*.

'I doubt very much whether this is a prophylactic procedure that Dr DeLee has described to us. He says he is going to prevent something. Unless he prevents something we are in fear of, I do not think he has made out a case for his operation... We have to remember that the number of women in hospitals is small; the majority of women are confined in their own homes under the care of general practitioners, and the technic of Dr DeLee is a hospital "stunt", and not one for the general practitioner... What is the matter, as a preventive, with properly sewing up the ordinary laceration which is so frequently found? If we taught students how to sew up these lacerations properly by vaginal stitching and taught them aseptic methods, in my opinion we would do more to prevent prolapse than by Dr DeLee's operation' (Eden, 1920:78).

The view that episiotomy was to be reserved for only 'abnormal' cases persisted during the 1920s. For example, in the first edition of *Queen Charlotte's Text-Book of Obstetrics* (Banister *et al.*, 1927), the description of episiotomy is found in the section of the book entitled 'Abnormal Labour'. In another text, *A Manual of Midwifery for Students and Practitioners* (Jellett & Madill, 1929), episiotomy was discussed in the chapter on 'Obstetrical Operations'.

During the 1930s, when American physicians were campaigning for the routine use of episiotomy on the grounds that it prevented or minimized the damage resulting from the alleged 'pathological' nature of childbirth, elements within the British medical establishment, in sharp contrast, continued to hold the view that childbirth was usually a normal process which should take place at home with as little intervention as possible. To quote the British Medical Association:

> '[birth is] a natural physiological event, though it is one involving complex, delicate and important processes. Departures from the normal occur in a small proportion of cases... All the available evidence demonstrates that normal confinements, and those which show a minor departure from normal, can be more safely conducted at home than in hospital' (British Medical Association, 1936:656).

In 1936 the British (later to become Royal) College of Obstetricians and Gynaecologists also supported this view, as the following excerpt from a British College of Obstetricians and Gynaecologists' memorandum on national maternity care indicates.

> '...adequate hospital provision for all cases could only be made at great expense: the results of domiciliary midwifery do not warrant such expenditure' (Campbell & Macfarlane, 1987, citing the British College of Obstetricians and Gynaecologists).

During the 1930s, the divergence of opinion between American and British physicians on the routine use of episiotomy was so strong that one particularly prominent London obstetrician felt compelled to speak out against his American colleagues' advocacy of the operation. During a 1936 talk on birth injuries (the prevention of which being one of the rationales offered by American obstetricians for performing episiotomy), Eardley Holland, Obstetric and Gynaecological Surgeon and Lecturer on Obstetrics and Gynaecology at London Hospital and co-author of *A Manual of Obstetrics* (Eden & Holland, 1937), told the AGS that 'prophylactic' episiotomy actually produced pathology rather than prevented it as the Americans claimed.

> 'The deep episiotomy is a disadvantage to a childbearing woman, in that it prevents her from losing the disadvantageous state of nulliparity as far as her pelvic floor and perineum are concerned' (Holland, 1936:59).

J.M. Munro Kerr, the eminent Scottish obstetrician (Emeritus Regius Professor of Midwifery at the University of Glasgow and Honorary Fellow of the Royal Society of Medicine in Ireland, the Edinburgh Obstetrical Society and the AGS), while accepting that episiotomy was beneficial when necessary, doubted it was often required. In the fourth edition of *Operative Obstetrics: A Guide to the Difficulties and Complications of Obstetric Practice*, Kerr (1937) writes:

'There is much to be said in its [episiotomy's] favour; it is much simpler to stitch accurately a clean incised lateral wound than a ragged one in the perineum. It is an operation, however, which is seldom necessary, provided the *accoucheur* attends to the points already referred to in the management of the perineum' (p.49).

In the next edition of his text, Kerr and his co-author Moir expanded the section on episiotomy. In their description of the operation in the chapter on intranatal care, they noted that 'some obstetricians, notably the late DeLee, have advised the routine use of episiotomy in all primigravidae' and countered this by stating:

'The chief objection to episiotomy is that every delivery is thereby converted into an operative procedure. The difficulty is to decide the cases in which episiotomy is required; for, on the one hand, if recourse is made to it too often it will be frequently performed unnecessarily, while on the other hand, if delayed too long any advantage to be gained in performing it will be lost. It is our opinion that, provided the *accoucheur* attends to the points already referred to, the operation is seldom necessary in a normal delivery' (Kerr & Moir, 1949:51).

In their chapter on operative obstetrics, Kerr and Moir further questioned the unnecessary use of the operation.

'The deliberate incision of the perineum – "prophylactic episiotomy" as it is sometimes termed – is now a common, perhaps too common, preliminary procedure to operative vaginal delivery. If prophylactic, it may be asked, prophylactic against what? And this brings us face to face with the question whether this operation, excellent in certain circumstances, is not, like so many other good methods of treatment, sometimes abused by being employed for trivial indications, and by operators who care little for the finer points of obstetric art...' (1949:852).

That British physicians rejected the use of episiotomy on the grounds that they believed 'normal delivery' did not produce sufficient damage to warrant elective episiotomy amazed American obstetricians. As one American physician observed after consulting Kerr and Moir's textbook:

'One of the outstanding examples of "preventive surgery" is the obstetrical episiotomy. This concept is not generally accepted since in Great Britain many object to "routine" episiotomy because it converts every delivery into an operative procedure...' (Savage, 1957:167).

During the 1950s, restricting the use of episiotomy in normal deliveries continued to be advised in British obstetrical textbooks, although the benefits claimed for the operation by American physicians were, nevertheless, also reported. For example, in the chapter 'Maternal Injuries' in the text *British Obstetric and Gynaecological Practice* edited by Holland and Bourne (1955), it was stated that:

'Episiotomy is thus highly prophylactic against utero-vaginal prolapse, stress incontinence, stillbirth, and the later effects of cerebral haemorrhage. Moreover, an incision is easier to repair than a laceration and heals better' (1955:785).

However, in the chapter entitled 'Management of Labour' they stated that 'this small operation is more frequently used for abnormal than for normal deliveries' (1955:147).

In the ninth edition of *Queen Charlotte's Text-Book of Obstetrics* (Gibberd *et al.*, 1956), episiotomy was suggested as a means of pre-empting an unavoidable perineal laceration because 'it has the advantage that a ragged tear or a tear involving the rectum are avoided, and it also prevents overstretching of the perineum which may subsequently be followed by prolapse' (Gibberd *et al.*, 1956:235). However, the text then goes on to state:

'Some authorities have advocated that episiotomy should be performed as a routine in every case. We do not favour this practice since it is unnecessary in a large number of cases, and because the patient is much more comfortable in the puerperium if perineal stitches can be avoided' (Beech, 1956:236).

Still other texts while acknowledging the benefits of episiotomy also raised concerns about the unnecessary use of the operation, as the following passages from *Practical Obstetrical Problems* by Donald (1955) indicate.

'The importance of this little operation is out of all proportion to its simplicity. Nevertheless, it is frequently abused. As an alternative injury to a second-degree tear its value is somewhat debatable, and to inflict a cut for no other reason than to prevent a tear is of dubious advantage, because the former may be more extensive than is actually necessary. Both, if properly sutured, heal equally well.

An episiotomy is infinitely preferable to an overstretched and devitalized perineum, with its parallel weakening of the supports of the bladder neck. Timely episiotomy can prevent a great deal of damage in this respect and is regarded as an important factor in the prevention of subsequent prolapse... The chief virtue of episiotomy lies in the saving of unnecessary wear and tear upon the foetal skull. This is particularly important in cases of prematurity.
... To withhold episiotomy when indicated would be wanton; never-

theless, it constitutes a mutilation, although mild, and if ruthlessly abused without good reason, it will leave a number of women exposed to the like-lihood of further perineal troubles in subsequent deliveries, often necessitating repeated episiotomy...' (pp. 421–2).

Although British national data on the use of episiotomy by physicians has never been collected, statistics from the 1958 British Perinatal Mortality Survey are suggestive of physicians' episiotomy rates. These data reveal that episiotomy was performed in only 21% of hospital births (most of these probably being performed by obstetricians or under their supervision) and in only 12% of births occurring in General Practitioner Units (small maternity units run by general practitioners usually with the assistance of midwives) (Anonymous, 1968:75).

Midwives and the restricted use of episiotomy

While there are no data on the use of episiotomy by midwives, the 1958 British Perinatal Mortality Survey reports that episiotomy was performed in only 2% of homebirths (the majority of homebirths being conducted by midwives, a minority by general practitioners). Clearly the midwifery philosophy that 'normal' cases should be left to nature promoted midwifery avoidance of episiotomy. Furthermore, the age-old midwifery practice of 'guarding' the perineum, considered by many as the hallmark of the midwifery expertise, discouraged its use in normal deliveries.

Perhaps the most important reason why midwives did not perform the operation was that they were actually prohibited from doing so by law. It was not until the summer of 1967 that the Central Midwives Board, the body governing the practice of midwifery in the UK, sanctioned for the first time the emergency use of episiotomy in normal births (Sleep, 1984a:29). While authorized to perform the operation, midwives were required to refer the repair of the incision to a medical practitioner. Midwives who had been taught the technique of repairing the perineum and were judged competent to do so could be authorized by a physician to carry out the procedure, although the responsibility for the perineal repair rested with the doctor (Arthure, 1970:1405). By requiring a medical officer to suture the incision, physicians retained their authority over the birth process and any midwife abusing the operation would be detected. For the same reason, repair of a perineal laceration has always been the responsibility of physicians. Until 1983, British midwives were required to seek a medical practitioner to suture perineal lacerations whenever they occurred (Sleep, 1984b:29).

Why the liberal use of episiotomy in the 1970s?

In contrast to the USA where the routinization of episiotomy was preceded by an intensive campaign to encourage the prophylactic use of episiotomy, in the UK no prominent obstetricians issued pleas in the periodical medical literature for the elective use of episiotomy. From time to time, individual obstetricians did advocate the prophylactic use of episiotomy (e.g. Salmond & Dearnley, 1935; Flew, 1944). For the most part, these were isolated appeals which failed to attract the interest of the profession.

The sudden popularity of episiotomy in the 1970s cannot be attributed to research demonstrating the alleged prophylactic benefits of the operation. Just as had been the case in the USA many decades earlier, the introduction of prophylactic episiotomy in the UK in the 1960s and 1970s occurred despite there being a total lack of scientific research showing the benefits or necessity of the operation. As Michael House, a Consultant Obstetrician Gynaecologist and Senior Lecturer in the Department of Obstetrics and Gynaecology at Charing Cross Hospital Medical School in London, reminded midwives in the early 1980s, 'it must be stressed at the outset that there is almost complete lack of any scientific evidence that the operation has any of the beneficial effects claimed for it' (House, 1981a:6).

The growing obstetrical use of episiotomy

Unlike in the USA and Canada where the routinization of episiotomy can be traced to an episiotomy campaign deliberately staged to promulgate the alleged benefits of the operation, in the UK the liberal use of episiotomy appears to have gradually crept into obstetric practice with little fanfare or notice. It seems the liberal use of episiotomy and the rationales supporting this practice were simply imported from the USA without much discussion in the medical literature. Childbirth activist Sheila Kitzinger described what happened in the following:

'... American obstetric practices tend to become British practices too, and after an interval of a few years become accepted as an integral part of our own "culture of childbirth". Interventionist obstetrics, of a kind which is now familiar in almost every British maternity unit, owe much of their origin to American practices' (Kitzinger, 1979a:233).

Evidence that the American claims about episiotomy were incorporated into British obstetric thought comes from what physicians were saying about the operation. As has been noted above, although indicating that the operation was seldom needed in normal deliveries, many of the most popular British obstetric textbooks from the 1930s onward claimed the same benefits of episiotomy as their American colleagues. This also occurred in the British periodical obstetrical literature where the American claims about prophylactic episiotomy benefits were reported.

> 'An episiotomy is infinitely preferable to an overstretched and deviated perineum, with its consequent and parallel weakening of the support of the bladder neck. A judiciously timed episiotomy can prevent a great deal of damage in this respect and is regarded by many as an important factor in the prevention of a prolapse of the uterus in later life' (Gunn, 1967:342).

The following comment by Michael House, Consultant Obstetrician at Charing Cross Hospital in London, confirms that the American claims about episiotomy were widely accepted by British physicians during the 1970s even though little direct evidence supported the claims.

> '... there is *no* evidence at all that episiotomies heal better than tears, which is one of the basic things which has been taught. I mean, as a student I was taught that episiotomies prevent tears, they're *better* in some divine way than tears, because doctors do them I suppose, and they heal better, they get less infection and they prevent prolapse. And really, there is no evidence for any of these statements at all. And I think most of the studies that have been done have backed this up. And I think it's, you know, it's spread ... it is one of those things that sort of crept in with no real evidence that it's of any benefit. But this is a common thing in medicine' (interview with Michael House).

The acceptance by some British physicians of the alleged prophylactic benefits of episiotomy is also apparent following the questioning of the elective use of episiotomy which became quite intense by the early 1980s. In coming to the defence of the practice, these physicians explicitly acknowledge their belief that episiotomy is prophylactic. For example, responding to an editorial on the growing elective use of episiotomy in the UK (Barker, 1981), Charles Flood, Senior Consultant in Obstetrics and Gynaecology at St George's and St James' Hospitals in London, replied by saying:

> 'Dr Barker seems to be completely unaware of the prime reason for performing an episiotomy and that is to preserve the tone and integrity of the perineal muscles. He states that there is a lack of acceptable evidence to support such claims as the prevention of prolapse, third degree tears and so on ... I do recall the late Sir Charles Read's comment, that whereas in the 1950s "repair of prolapse" was the commonest major operation on gynaecological waiting lists in the United Kingdom, when he went to America and was asked to demonstrate a Fothergill's operation, his American colleagues had great difficulty in finding a patient upon whom he could operate!' (Flood, 1982:51)

Similar views can also be found in letters to the editor of the *British Medical Journal* (e.g. Crawford, 1982; Hodgkin, 1982).

An examination of successive editions of *Munro Kerr's Operative Obstetrics* and Dewhurst's *Integrated Obstetrics and Gynaecology for Postgraduates* confirms that a shift in British obstetricians' attitudes about episiotomy occurred sometime between the early 1960s and 1980s, which corresponds with the data on the rate of episiotomy in England and Wales during these years. For example, while the seventh edition of *Munro Kerr's Operative Obstetrics* published in 1964 objected to the liberal use of episiotomy, this was not the case in the eighth edition published in 1971 as the following passage reveals:

> 'The late DeLee of Chicago was among the first to advocate routine epi-siotomy in all primiparae, but the more conservatively-minded obste-tricians in this country were in general opposed to the idea of converting a "normal" into an "operative" delivery. In the intervening years opinion has steadily turned in its favour, and personally I use it [mid-line epi-siotomy] for all cases in which the foetus is large or even average in size, or in which the vulvar introitus is unnecessarily tight' (Moir & Myers-cough, 1971:27).

A similar shift is also evident between the 1976 and 1981 edition of Dewhurst's *Integrated Obstetrics and Gynaecology for Postgraduates*. In the second edition of this text published in 1976, Dewhurst simply stated that episiotomy 'is most frequently done in primigravida and in hos-pital practice for a variety of reasons' and then goes on to list eight indications for the operation along with the method of performing the operation. In the third edition of the text, the section on episiotomy was rewritten and included for the first time the following sentences, 'The modern *accoucheur* simply looks for reasons why an episiotomy should not be performed. There are few' (Dewhurst, 1981:456).

The sudden and dramatic increase in the use of episiotomy in the UK resulted from a number of circumstances. Some of these prompted physicians to perform the operation more often, while others acted to encourage its use by midwives. Unfortunately, as there are no data differentiating the medical from midwifery use of episiotomy, it is impossible to know the precise impact each set of factors had on increased use.

As for the reason for this change, some have suggested that the increasing popularity of episiotomy simply resulted from the growing proportion of births taking place in hospital. As a 1968 editorial in the *Lancet* speculated:

> 'Eastman pointed out that it was the shift from home to hospital confinement in the United States which offered doctors better facilities and encouraged them to perform episiotomy more often. With the increase in hospital con-

finements in the United Kingdom a similar trend may become apparent' (Anonymous, 1968:75).

The move to hospital births with the availability of 'hospital facilities' (i.e. technology) does appear to have been associated with the increasing use of episiotomy by physicians and midwives. Assuming about 65% of births took place in hospital in 1958 (Campbell & Macfarlane, 1987:12) and an episiotomy rate in hospital of 21% (Anonymous, 1968), the episiotomy rate for all births in 1958 would have been at least 14% (this is a conservative estimate as this calculation ignores episiotomies performed in general practitioner units and at home-births). By 1968 when the *Lancet* editorial was written, the percentage of births taking place in hospital had risen by about 15% to 80.6% (Campbell & Macfarlane, 1987:12), and the national episiotomy rate had risen by approximately 10% to 25% (Macfarlane & Mugford, 1984:245). Since only physicians were permitted to perform the operation prior to 1967, the increase in the episiotomy rate is directly attributable to increased use by physicians.

Between 1968 and 1978, the proportion of births in hospital rose by another 17% (increasing from 80.6% to 97.1%). The national episiotomy rate during this period more than doubled, increasing by over 28% (rising from 25% to 53.4% of all births). While the use of episiotomy was associated with the increase in hospital births, the increasing use of the operation during the period when the percentage of hospital births had stabilized suggests that factors in addition to the increase in hospital births also played a role in the growing popularity of the operation.

Induction of labour and the 'active management of labour'

During the early 1970s, both the practice of medically inducing labour and the 'active management of labour' began to firmly take hold. Induction is the process of electively initiating labour and keeping it going whereas the active management of labour (O'Driscoll *et al.*, 1973; O'Driscoll & Meagher, 1980) involves augmenting or stimulating labour which has begun spontaneously. Both practices are methods of conducting childbirth so as to minimize the length of time a woman is in labour, although the stages of active management of labour have been clearly defined.

For women giving birth for the first time, active management of labour involves artificial rupture of the membranes (ARM) which is performed within one hour of the onset of labour to speed up the dilatation of the cervix. One hour later, the process is further speeded up with the intravenous administration of oxytocin (O'Driscoll &

Meagher, 1980). Under this model, no labour is allowed to last longer than 12 hours. Active management of labour is another example of an unevaluated procedure which was undertaken and enthusiastically copied elsewhere with no evidence of benefit when used routinely.

Although national data on the use of active management of labour are not available, the percentage of labours induced more than doubled in seven years, from 16.8% of all labours in 1967 to 38.9% in 1974 (Fig. 4). These data would seem to support Oakley's (1986) observation that improvements in the safety and efficacy of pharmacologically initiated labour since the 1950s made it 'possible for obstetricians to broaden the indications for induction to include many pregnancies which 50 or 20 years before would have been regarded as normal and inappropriate candidates for artificial induction' (p. 206). The use of episiotomy was not an explicit component of elective induction or the obstetrical package known as active management of labour. Yet as had been the case with the 'prophylactic forceps operation' of the 1920s, episiotomy was nevertheless indirectly encouraged. The growing use of induction initiated a 'cascade of intervention' (Inch, 1984), which led to the presumed necessity of performing episiotomy. Kitzinger, considered the Dean of childbirth education, describes the process in the following way:

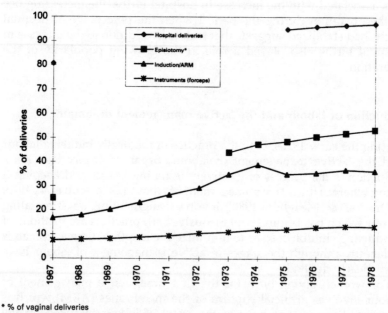

* % of vaginal deliveries
Source: Macfarlane & Mugford, 1984:245.

Fig. 4   Changes in obstetrical practices in England and Wales (1967–1978).

'It seems to me that one could see a parallel ... I don't know whether it is cause and effect or not, but once you start inducing labours ... and of course remember in Britain in the early 70s, nearly half of all labours were induced. Once you start inducing labours and then, if you are not inducing them, augmenting them, you are actually pushing a baby down with a strongly contracting uterus before all the tissues have fanned out and the woman's body is really ready for that baby to be pushed out. And so I think what often happens is, and I have observed this sitting watching labours in hospitals, I've seen a drip set up, an intravenous drip, a uterus contracting strongly, *down* comes the head and then they do an episiotomy because they get a shiny almost white perineum looking like a balloon about to pop' (interview with Sheila Kitzinger).

A study of obstetrical practices in the Oxford area between 1965 and 1972 documents what Kitzinger and others (e.g. Massey & Bates, 1975; Adamson, 1978) suspected. The increasing use of episiotomy was in part attributable to a cascade of intervention which was initiated by the induction of labour. In this study (Fedrick & Yudkin, 1976:738), episiotomy was found to be 'twice as prevalent in induced as in non-induced cases'.

While the rising rate of induction may have encouraged the use of episiotomy in some cases, this too is only a partial explanation. As indicated in Fig. 4, throughout this period (1967–1978), the episiotomy rate exceeded the induction rate. Furthermore, the induction rate peaked in 1974 at 38.9% and then dropped, levelling off at about 35% from 1975 to 1978. For the most part, the decrease in the use of induction resulted from a nationwide debate concerning the widespread use of induction in normal labour (Anonymous, 1974 ; Chalmers, 1976a; interview with Iain Chalmers). Had the increasing episiotomy rate been solely related to the use of induction, both interventions should have shown similar declines. Since the episiotomy rate has always been higher than the induction rate and continued to climb despite the reduction in induced labours, factors other than induction were also important in bringing about the liberal use of episiotomy.

Figure 4 also reveals that the rising episiotomy rate appears not to have been correlated with the rate of instrumental delivery (forceps) as it was in the USA so many years earlier.

Midwifery use of episiotomy

The rapid assimilation of episiotomy into midwifery practice in the UK resulted from both the lifting of the Central Midwives Board regulation which had barred midwives from performing perineal incision, and the almost complete integration of midwifery into hospital practice during the early 1970s (Robinson *et al.*, 1983). Following the authorization of midwives to perform emergency episiotomy in 1967 and the release of the 1970 Peel Report recommending that all births take place in hospital, both the episiotomy rate and the proportion of births taking place in hospital increased sharply. As one consultant obstetrician and gynaecologist observed in 1973, 'it is an operation which is being left more and more to midwives to perform ... In fact it is becoming an important midwife's operation' (Beynon, 1973:25).

Data from the West Middlesex Hospital in London indicate that the increasing use of episiotomy was directly related to the shift from community to hospital midwifery. In the early 1970s, this hospital, like many others in the UK, set up a system known as the 'domino' scheme to integrate community midwifery into hospital practice. Domino is an acronym for domiciliary in and out of hospital. Under this scheme, community midwives taking care of 'normal' or low risk women would, at the onset of labour, accompany their clients into hospital and take responsibility for the delivery. If there were no complications, the women could go home within a few hours after the delivery.

When the domino scheme was first set up in 1971, the episiotomy rate for the hospital was 40%, rising to 55% by 1977. The episiotomy rate for domino cases for these years was 4% and 38% respectively. When the programme first started, the domiciliary midwives were performing episiotomy at the same rate as they had at home births (4%). Within six years of working within the hospital system, their use of episiotomy had increased eight-fold and was nearing the episiotomy rate found in the hospital when the domino scheme started.

At the time, the explanation given for the domino midwives' rapid adoption of episiotomy was that being in hospital, the midwives now had ready access to the physicians who could immediately suture episiotomy incisions and were now required to follow the consultant's policies. In contrast, at homebirths, a major impediment to midwives performing the operation was having to call for a physician to repair an episiotomy incision after the delivery. As the Honorary Consultant Obstetrician and Gynaecologist to the West Middlesex Hospital pointed out at the time:

'Prior to this [the introduction of the domino scheme], as domiciliary midwives, they were dependent on general practitioners for perineal suturing. The doctor's availability was subsequently affected by other commitments, and the prospect of a long wait for their mothers discouraged a more liberal use of episiotomy. Now, with immediate access to a doctor's services in the delivery suite for those midwives who prefer not to undertake perineal repairs, the episiotomy rate is approaching that found in the overall obstetric population' (Fox, 1979:337-8).

As described above, the availability of facilities and technology in hospitals in the USA encouraged the routine use of episiotomy. In a similar fashion, community midwives in the UK who were becoming integrated into hospital practice and midwives already working in hospitals probably also found the hospital environment encouraged the liberal use of the operation. No doubt, midwives found both the 'operating-room' conditions in hospital and the availability of physicians who could immediately suture an episiotomy incision conducive to performing the operation. In addition to the availability of hospital facilities and personnel, other factors related to midwifery autonomy and local practice norms also helped accelerate the liberal use of episiotomy.

The loss of autonomy of hospital midwives

As more and more midwives began working in hospitals, they found themselves within an organizational structure which limited, and in many cases greatly diminished, their autonomy and ability to assist in labours as they saw fit. Where domiciliary midwives accepted total responsibility for the homebirths and sought medical attention only when a particular case warranted it, hospital midwives came under the direct supervision and direction of consultant obstetricians. As Robinson (1990) noted, during the 1960s and 1970s medical staff became increasingly involved in normal maternity care while the freedom of midwives to exercise clinical judgement diminished. Mary Renfrew (Chair of Midwifery at the University of Leeds and former midwifery researcher at the National Perinatal Epidemiology Unit, Oxford) and Michael House (Consultant Obstetrician Gynaecologist, Charing Cross Hospital Medical School, London) explain how the assimilation of midwives into hospital practice impacted on their activities during labour and delivery:

> 'You are quite right to target the Peel Report because up until that point, if you like, midwives were very much in charge of what they did at delivery. Because a lot of what was going on was at home, even in hospital, there was not a lot of intervention or doctors in births where midwives were in charge. And you know that in this country [the UK], I mean even nowadays, at almost 70% of births, the midwife is the senior person present, there isn't actually a doctor physically present in the room unless they're needed for instrumental births. And so the midwife, certainly let's talk about up until the time of the Peel Report and the *move* from home into hospital, was very much in charge of what was happening and was carrying out traditional midwifery practice which was episiotomy when necessary, but generally trying to have an intact perineum. Once everything began to get more and more hospitalized, interventions were easier for the obstetricians to impose. I

mean, I think electronic fetal monitoring is part of that picture and the other things that were possible because of hospitalization. And episiotomy rose dramatically during that time. And when I trained as a midwife in 1978, it was never questioned but every first-time mother had an episiotomy. That was how I was taught in 1978 by midwives. So what you saw from the 1960s through into the 1970s was an increase in routine intervention that midwives simply took on board for a while, although there were movements against it, but for a while, I think, it swept over the midwifery profession very fast' (interview with Mary Renfrew).

'... you know what happened was, there was a change in sort of emphasis on obstetric care which is now swinging the other way. The pendulum is going across. Basically ... there was a real swing from midwives being ... sort of the primary carers and obstetricians dealing with the problems, like when I was a student perhaps 20 or 30 years ago, to all of it being not midwifery. When I was a student, the textbooks were called textbooks of midwifery and then it changed to obstetrics. And there was a big change in emphasis you know, *doctors* were now in charge. And midwives, basically their role became degraded down to obstetric nurses. This was another thing I thought was a very *bad* move. And as a result of this, I think because obstetricians are basically surgeons and they for some reason or other convinced themselves that episiotomies were good, this tremendous upswing in episiotomies occurred. And as I said already, with obstetricians saying that tears were bad, midwives started to copy them' (interview with Michael House).

Local norms of practice: maternity unit and midwifery training policies

As Renfrew and House suggest, physicians largely influenced hospital midwifery practice through both informal and formal means. Informally, physicians established and reinforced local 'norms' which promoted the liberal use of episiotomy by midwives. One such norm relates to the intolerance consultant obstetricians held for perineal lacerations. Many consultant obstetricians had come to believe the American claims that episiotomies prevent perineal lacerations, are easier to repair and heal better than a spontaneous tear. The following passages suggest that such norms existed in some maternity units. The quotations are taken from letters written by consultant obstetricians and gynaecologists in response to a 1980 survey of obstetrical units conducted by House.

'In general terms I am quite prepared to make the statement that perineal tears occur in my unit infrequently as the staff *know* how much better it is to repair a clean episiotomy and carry it out when a tear can be foreseen' (House, privileged correspondence).

'I think it reasonable to state that our policy would be that we would prefer to carry out a controlled episiotomy than an uncontrolled tear' (House, privileged correspondence).

In units where this view predominated, a perineal tear, even a small one, was often considered evidence of poor delivery technique, while performing an episiotomy was absolutely acceptable (Levett, 1974; Fisher, 1981). Under these circumstances, many midwives tended to opt for performing an episiotomy to avoid the occurrence of a perineal laceration and the reprimand that would have gone along with it. The following passage from a community midwife describes how this 'local norm' affected many midwives in the 1970s and early 1980s.

'...in hospital, where episiotomies are so much the norm, it becomes an absolute disgrace on the midwives' part to allow a perineum to tear – even a small nick which requires no suturing is considered a mark of gross ineffi- ciency. Thus, as a young midwife or a pupil, one becomes so terrified of allowing a perineum to tear that to do a routine episiotomy becomes the easiest answer – no one is ever criticized for an unnecessary episiotomy!' (Levett, 1974:89)

House offers a similar interpretation of what occurred during the 1970s.

'Midwives didn't like doing episiotomies. But the reason they did so many, is for years they have been rapped on the knuckles, metaphorically speaking, for *allowing* tears to happen. So their response, well if you say episiotomy prevents tears, and I know I'm never going to get told off for doing an episiotomy, I'll do episiotomies. And so it crept up. That's the reason, I'm absolutely sure. Obstetricians say tears are bad, episiotomies are good. That went down the line to the midwives and they started doing a lot but they didn't like doing it' (interview with Michael House).

As midwives at one hospital pointed out, a major stimulus for doing an episiotomy was the 'ignominy of calling a registrar [resident] for a third degree tear because an episiotomy was not performed in time' (Barker, 1981:41).

Consultant obstetricians also influenced midwifery use of epi- siotomy by setting formal maternity unit policies and protocols. Although a 1984 survey of English Health Districts (Garcia & Garforth, 1989) failed to reveal any written maternity unit policies requiring routine episiotomy, the results of House's survey suggest such policies, while perhaps not explicitly documented, were nonetheless operating in some hospitals. The survey reveals huge variations in the rates of episiotomy with the rate for primigravidae and multiparae ranging from 14% to 96% and 16% to 71% respectively (House *et al.*, 1986). As the following passage indicates, some midwives were well aware of the role unit policies played in their increased use of episiotomy.

'Presumably the incidence of episiotomy is largely determined by obstetric unit policy ... Left to themselves and to their own judgement, however, there are certainly those midwives who would be far more reluctant to resort to the scissors than at present were they not obliged to bow to a higher authority' (Dixon, 1981).

In a few cases, midwives have even been ordered to perform the operation in normal deliveries. In at least one documented case, such an order resulted in a midwife performing an episiotomy after the delivery because she had not had time to do it before (Robinson, 1982). Beverley Lawrence Beech, Honorary Chair of the AIMS, a maternity pressure group, tells of other cases of which she has personal knowledge where midwives were told to do episiotomies and 'had been carpeted by the consultant for not doing an episiotomy' (interview with Beverley Lawrence Beech). In most cases, however, it is more likely that midwives simply deferred to the consultant obstetrician's favourable opinion of elective episiotomy. Because the consultant obstetrician is at the pinnacle of the maternity unit hierarchy, midwives simply accepted what the consultant said about the prophylactic benefits of episiotomy and followed their wishes. As Caroline Flint, consultant in maternity and child health, author of a midwifery textbook and past president of the Royal College of Midwives points out, the power differential between midwives and obstetricians made midwives vulnerable to the consultant's pronouncements about elective episiotomy.

'Obstetricians are very self-confident and they expect people to do what they say. And so you have midwives going, you know, hearing what ... these very important, powerful men were saying, [with an upper class British accent] "Episiotomies. We need to do episiotomies. We can't let these poor women suffer. Their pelvic floors will be destroyed". And the midwife says [lowering her voice and sounding diminutive and respectful], "Alright. Yes sir, yes sir". You know, and no midwife ever thought, is there any research justification? She would no more challenge this great man than fly to the moon' (interview with Caroline Flint).

Another maternity unit protocol which midwives (Dixon, 1981; Fisher, 1981; Wilkerson, 1984), childbirth activists and childbearing women (Adamson, 1978) have identified as encouraging the use of episiotomy relates to the setting of time limits on the second stage of labour. In some cases, these protocols required midwives to call an obstetrician to perform a forceps delivery when the allowable time limit had expired. To avoid a forceps delivery, midwives would perform an episiotomy to facilitate and hasten the labour. In the following passage, Chloe Fisher, then Senior Nursing Officer for Community Midwifery at the Oxford Radcliffe NHS Trust Hospital, describes how the integration of midwives into hospital practice and the obstetrical imposition of time limits on labour influenced the midwifery use of episiotomy.

'During the last twenty years or so the percentage of women giving birth in hospitals with obstetricians in charge has risen enormously. Previously they had been the responsibility of midwives and general practitioners either at home or in small cottage hospital-type general practitioner units. During this time the permissible duration of the second stage for primigravida has become shorter and shorter – even to as little as thirty minutes. A major reason for this increase in episiotomies, therefore, has been the midwife's attempt to enable the woman in her care to achieve a spontaneous delivery in the limited time allowed – knowing that otherwise she must hand her delivery over to the obstetrician to be delivered by forceps' (Fisher, 1981:12).

Another policy which probably encouraged the use of episiotomy related to midwifery training requirements. Although not required by the National Board, during the 1970s, individual midwifery schools often required student midwives to carry out a specified number of the operations during their training. For example, one midwifery school required all its students to perform ten episiotomies before qualifying. The number of episiotomies students had to perform during their training varied between midwifery schools and these 'policies' were seldom, if ever, written down.

The pressures on the ward

Finally, one other factor that played a role in the increasing reliance on episiotomy by midwives was the hospital work environment. When midwives attended women in their homes, they had only one patient to care for, there were no arbitrary time limits set on the length of the second stage, and they could provide continuity of care (they stayed with the woman throughout the delivery). All of these factors help develop the relationship between the midwife and the woman, making it much less likely the midwife would need to resort to episiotomy. As one community midwife has noted:

'... the nurse–patient relationship at home is often very much better by this stage of labour than in hospital (because of hospital staff changes, of duty, etc.) so the home midwife is much more able to rely on maximum co-operation from the mother at crowning, and so ensure slow delivery of a well-flexed vertex and thus minimal damage to the perineum (Levett, 1974:89).

On a busy maternity unit with staff changing at each shift, a midwife who might be caring for several women simultaneously approaching second stage crowning, might not be able to assure a slow unhurried second stage, the very conditions needed to avoid an episiotomy. These conditions can contribute to the more liberal use of episiotomy by midwives by interfering with the midwife–patient relationship and by causing midwives to be overworked. When the midwife–patient relationship is less well developed, the patient is less able to co-operate with the midwife during the birth as described above by Levett.

Caring for several women at the same time places pressure on a midwife to deliver each woman as quickly as possible so as to be able to attend to the next expectant mother who is waiting for her. Observational data from the Royal Berkshire Hospital in Reading would seem to support this. As Sleep, a midwifery researcher explains, 'the busier the labour ward is, the more episiotomies are done. If you've got a very busy month, you get a high episiotomy rate, if you get a slower month, you get a lower one' (interview with Jennifer Sleep). This observation has been made by other midwives as well (Wilkerson, 1984). In the following passage, Sleep elaborates on the pressure hospital midwives experience on a busy maternity unit and the importance of their having the confidence to resist performing an episiotomy under these conditions.

'Midwives have just got to stick with it, they've just got to maintain that confidence that they can deliver with minimal intervention and then it's alright to not be hassled by somebody else saying, "Well come on hurry up". You know, "we need ... we've got people waiting for this room" or "you need to be next door because there is somebody else advanced there and we haven't got another member of the staff to look after her", or whatever' (interview with Jennifer Sleep).

Chapter 5

The Challenging of Obstetric Orthodoxy in the UK

Despite the rapid and steady increase in the use of episiotomy during the 1970s in the UK, this trend levelled off and reversed in the early 1980s. As graphically presented in Fig. 3 within seven years (1978–1985) the national episiotomy rate in England declined from 53.4% to 36.6%, an absolute and relative reduction of 17% and 31% respectively. This chapter primarily examines the events and activities that led to the practice of routine episiotomy losing favour in England during the early 1980s.

The rise of professional questioning of episiotomy

Concerns about the increasing popularity of episiotomy and lack of evidence of the benefits of the operation were raised early on in the medical literature by J.K. Russell in an anonymous leading article in the *Lancet* (Anonymous, 1968). Russell, Professor of Obstetrics and Gynaecology at the University of Newcastle-upon-Tyne, was prompted to write the leading article by the high incidence of episiotomy he witnessed as a Visiting Professor at Louis Hellman's obstetrical unit in New York in 1967 and by 'intense discussions/arguments about all aspects of episiotomy' he had with American colleagues: Hellman and Nicholson Eastman (authors of the thirteenth edition of *Williams Obstetrics*) and Hellman's friends, John Parks and Robert Barter (Russell, personal communication). The intent of the leading article was to make physicians think about the immediate and long-term implications of episiotomy. However, with the exception of one obstetric textbook which described Russell's leading article (Beazley, 1986), it does not appear to have provoked a response in the periodical literature.

More questions were raised about episiotomy in early 1974 in a letter in response to an editorial on pain after childbirth published in the *British Medical Journal* (BMJ) (Anonymous, 1973). Robyn Pogmore, an Australian trained physician who was living in England, bitterly complained that midwives and obstetricians showed little interest in perineal pain after birth. She referred to episiotomy as 'deliberate mutilation of the maternal perineum', and challenged the widely accepted rationale that episiotomy prevented perineal lacerations. She also identified post-episiotomy pain as a serious problem for many women.

'I think that episiotomies are performed much too freely. They do not necessarily prevent tearing and the wound is hideously painful for weeks afterwards, and maybe for years' (Pogmore, 1974:37).

As Pogmore herself predicted, her letter failed to provoke any comment or discussion in the *BMJ* about the benefits of episiotomy or its increasing use. It did, however, prompt two letters which attempted to explain the reasons for postpartum perineal pain rather than question the practice of episiotomy as Pogmore had done. One letter by J. Chassar Moir, Emeritus Professor of Obstetrics and Gynaecology at Oxford University and author of several editions of *Munro Kerr's Operative Obstetrics*, suggested that the type of episiotomy performed was related to the amount of perineal discomfort women experienced (Chassar Moir, 1974). The other letter blamed the method of suturing perineal incisions as the cause of much post-episiotomy pain (Morris, 1974).

Midwifery questioning of the practice appeared for the first time in 1974 when Dinah Levett, a midwife and antenatal (prenatal) teacher for the National Childbirth Trust (NCT), published a one page polemical report on episiotomy in *Nursing Mirror* (Levett, 1974). In the article, Levett noted that the operation had become almost routine in hospital births and questioned the alleged benefits of episiotomy in preventing tears and prolapse. This article, like earlier medical questioning of episiotomy, failed to encourage broader midwifery questioning of episiotomy.

In 1975, Iain Chalmers, a Medical Research Fellow in the Department of Medical Statistics at the Welsh National School of Medicine, observed that despite the increasing use of episiotomy in the country, the tear rate had not been significantly reduced as would be expected had the claim that episiotomy prevents tears been true (Chalmers, 1975). Additional concern about episiotomy which also appears to have been to no avail came in 1976 with Chalmers' advocacy of evidence-based perinatal medicine (Chalmers, 1976a). In a paper published in the journal *Pediatrics*, Chalmers called on researchers to conduct randomized controlled trials (RCTs) to evaluate new and widely accepted perinatal practices. He noted that episiotomy was one of the many maternity practices for which there was little scientific data showing circumstances under which the operation was beneficial. In the years to come, Chalmers would have a monumental impact on the challenging of episiotomy by encouraging the questioning of all obstetrical practices as Director of the National Perinatal Epidemiology Unit in Oxford.

It was not until three years later in 1979 that the concerted and repeated questioning of episiotomy began. Juliet Willmott, a community midwife, noted in *Nursing Mirror* that routine episiotomy was the 'latest craze' in some obstetrics departments (1979:31). Referring to the idea of routine episiotomy as 'atrocious', Willmott questioned the alleged prophylactic benefits of the operation. She took particular exception to the obstetrical theory 'that women have an in-built pelvic flaw which makes it imperative to do an episiotomy' (1979:31). In February of 1980, Willmott published a second critique, this time in *Midwives Chronicle and Nursing Notes*, the official journal of the Royal College of Midwives. Willmott reiterated her earlier concerns about the indiscriminate use of episiotomy which appeared to be taking place in many hospitals. Based on her own clinical experience, she disputed the 'irresponsible medical propaganda' about the prophylactic benefits of episiotomy.

In early 1981, more controversy about the operation was generated within the midwifery profession by Norman Morris, editor of *Midwife, Health Visitor and Community Nurse*. Morris, who was Professor of Obstetrics and Gynaecology at London University at Charing Cross Hospital Medical School and also Deputy Vice Chancellor of London University and President of the Royal Society of Medicine's section on Obstetrics and Gynaecology, opened the January issue of his journal with an editorial questioning the scientific basis for the frequent use of episiotomy. He ended the editorial by challenging obstetric units to re-examine their use of the practice (Morris, 1981).

Morris' editorial was immediately followed by a review of the episiotomy literature by Michael House, a consultant obstetrician gynaecologist at Morris' hospital. In reviewing the literature, House found little evidence to support the claims made for routinely performing the operation and called for a complete reappraisal of the whole matter 'in the hope that a drastic reduction in the incidence of this "minor" operation can be achieved in the future' (House, 1981a:9). House's article prompted several letters to the journal which expressed gratitude that someone of the stature of a consultant obstetrician was seriously questioning the practice of routine episiotomy (e.g. Bromwich, 1981; Dixon, 1981). It was also around this same time that House began inquiring about the episiotomy rate in all the maternity units in the UK. The many hostile responses House received would seem to suggest that many maternity units across the country were unprepared at this time to seriously question their unit's policies regarding the use of episiotomy (interview with

Michael House; personal communication (responses to House's 1980 survey of maternity units)).

While debate within midwifery about the value of routine episiotomy began developing in 1979, the same thing did not occur within the medical literature until a senior registrar in obstetrics and gynaecology published a one page critique in *World Medicine* in August 1981 (Barker, 1981). The article drew attention to the developing divergence of professional opinion concerning the need for, or benefits of, routine episiotomy. A large part of the article was devoted to presenting House's views on episiotomy.

By January 1982, the medical controversy over the routine use of episiotomy intensified greatly with the publication of a second editorial by Professor Russell, this time signed, in the *British Medical Journal* (Russell, 1982). Concerned that the use of episiotomy may have been getting out of hand, Russell, now the Dean of Postgraduate Medicine at the University of Newcastle-upon-Tyne, acknowledged that there were few objective data to support the benefits claimed for episiotomy. Attention was further focused on episiotomy with the publication of an uncontrolled prospective study of post-episiotomy pain which appeared in the same issue of the *BMJ* (Reading *et al.*, 1982). The study of 101 women offered evidence that episiotomy was associated with high levels of pain, in many cases persisting for up to three months. At three months postpartum, one-third of women reported having had a problem with the episiotomy repair that required them to seek professional help.

In the subsequent four issues of the *BMJ*, an interactive debate over episiotomy erupted; no less than a dozen letters were published which either questioned or defended the practice (Beynon, 1982; Cockersell, 1982; Crawford, 1982; Garrey, 1982; Hodgkin, 1982; Kitzinger, 1982; Lau, 1982; Lee, 1982; Polden, 1982; Pretorius, 1982; Reading, 1982; Woinarski, 1982).

In February 1982, discussion about routine episiotomy continued in the medical literature when Charles Flood, a Senior Consultant in Obstetrics and Gynaecology at St George's and St James' Hospitals (London) and Vice President of the South West London Obstetrical Society, replied to Barker's critique of episiotomy in *World Medicine* (Flood, 1982). Flood chastized Barker for seemingly being 'completely unaware ... [that] the prime reason for performing an episiotomy ... [was] to preserve the tone and integrity of the perineal muscles' (Flood, 1982:51). He also supported the view that episiotomy prevented uterine and vaginal prolapse by pointing to the lower incidence of these conditions in the USA where 'practically every primigravida patient has an episiotomy' (p. 51).

By the summer of 1982, questioning of episiotomy by physicians and midwives had become so significant that the first two RCTs to scientifically evaluate the alleged prophylactic benefits of episiotomy were mounted (Harrison *et al.*, 1984; Sleep *et al.*, 1984). An RCT is an experiment in which subjects are randomly allocated to receive one particular treatment or approach. The RCT is considered the gold standard in medical research because its experimental design minimizes the possibility of bias. It is only undertaken at that point when controversy over a particular treatment or practice is so great that many clinicians become uncertain as to the most appropriate action to take. If something is known to work (and to be acceptable and without harmful effects), then there is no reason to submit it to this form of clinical trial. For these reasons, the very mounting of the episiotomy RCTs signifies that the practice of episiotomy must have, by this time, become quite controversial within midwifery and obstetrics.

During the summer of 1982, controversy over routine episiotomy continued when general practitioners were brought into the debate by Luke Zander (1982) with an editorial in the *Journal of the Royal College of General Practitioners* entitled 'Episiotomy: has familiarity bred contempt?'. Zander, an ex-president of the General Practice section of the Royal Society of Medicine and Senior Lecturer in the Department of General Practice at St Thomas' Hospital in London, called for a whole reappraisal of the conduct of labour, including the use of episiotomy. In the autumn of 1982, discussions about routine episiotomy persisted in the midwifery literature, this time with respect to the issue of informed consent (Finch, 1982). Midwives were cautioned by a barrister that an episiotomy performed routinely or which was opposed by a client was tantamount to battery.

The following year, questioning of episiotomy by midwives continued with the publication of results of a small unrepresentative survey on tears and episiotomies (Needham & Sheriff, 1983). The study, while not generalizable, undermined some of the traditional rationales for performing the operation. The midwifery investigators concluded that 'a perineal tear heals and is far more comfortable than episiotomy', and that patients experiencing problems were more likely to be those who had had an episiotomy. In April, medicolegal issues relating to the routine use of episiotomy were revisited in the midwifery literature. Midwives were counselled to obtain maternity patients' consent for all procedures, even routine ones such as episiotomy, and warned that '... performing episiotomy without adequate consent is a serious offence and is an act which could open up the possibility of an action for heavy damages against those involved' (Finch, 1983). Also during 1983 House initiated a third episiotomy RCT in London (House *et al.*, 1986).

In 1984, results of the episiotomy RCTs began appearing in the professional literature. In January, Jennifer Sleep (1984a), principal investigator of the West Berkshire episiotomy trial, reported preliminary analysis of the study in the journal *Nursing*. She also stated that the data suggested that 'the liberal use of episiotomy was unjustified in terms of minimizing trauma, reducing pain (including dyspareunia – difficult painful sexual intercourse) and improved healing after delivery' (Sleep, 1984a·614)

Still more questioning of episiotomy occurred with the publication in *Midwives Chronicle and Nursing Notes* of a retrospective study of episiotomy rates from one obstetric unit. Valerie Wilkerson, a hospital midwifery sister, studied the episiotomy rate of 21 midwives. She found huge variations between midwives, suggesting that the use of episiotomy, at least in her hospital, was not rational. Observing the lack of consistency in performing the operation, she concluded that '...the likelihood of episiotomy is apparently determined, not by the condition of the mother or baby, but by which midwife is allocated to the case' (Wilkerson, 1984:109). Wilkerson called on the advocates of episiotomy to justify the claims made for it and, until evidence was offered, she instructed midwives to 'again seek to establish the intact perineum as one of the hallmarks' of midwifery skill (p.109).

By the summer of 1984, the scientific evidence from RCTs was mounting against the routine use of episiotomy. Data from the Dublin and West Berkshire trials indicated that the routine or liberal use of episiotomy was unjustified. Neither trial produced evidence to support the alleged prophylactic benefits of episiotomy – that it minimized perineal trauma, reduced postpartum pain, or improved perineal healing after delivery. Based on their results, the researchers of both trials called for the abandonment of the practice of routine episiotomy. The results from the Dublin trial were the first to be published in the 30 June issue of the *BMJ* (Harrison *et al.*, 1984), followed shortly thereafter by the publication of the results of the West Berkshire trial in the 8 September issue (Sleep *et al.*, 1984). Summaries of the results of the West Berkshire trial were also published by Sleep (1984a;c) in the nursing literature. In addition, the results of the West Berkshire trial were also widely disseminated at midwifery conferences and study days before and after being published.

Controversy over episiotomy continued to be fuelled with the publication of other observational episiotomy studies in 1984; one by a midwife (Carter, 1984), and another by a general practice trainee and a consultant obstetrician (Jackson & Dunster, 1984). At the same time, another non-evidence-based criticism also appeared in the medical literature (McCullough, 1984).

In 1985, the last year for which there are national episiotomy statistics, discussion of episiotomy declined substantially from the flurry of activity in 1984. One non-evidence-based critique of episiotomy appeared in the midwifery literature (Flint, 1985). Also, one controlled non-randomized study was published which disputed the claim that episiotomy prevented pelvic relaxation (Gordon & Logue, 1985). The authors concluded that the study failed 'to support the theory that episiotomy results in improved healing and better perineal muscle function, and there is no evidence to suggest that an intact perineum in childbirth gives rise to deficient function due to over-stretching'.

A Belgian observational study published in the *British Journal of Obstetrics and Gynaecology* in August 1985 (Buekens *et al.*, 1985) addressed the relationship between episiotomy and third-degree tears. British obstetricians often offered prevention of third-degree perineal lacerations as the rationale for performing episiotomy. Contrary to physician belief, the study of nearly 22 000 births found no relation between episiotomy and third-degree tears after stratifying the data by birthweight and parity. Additional questions of the value of episiotomy in preventing third-degree tears appeared in an October editorial in the *Lancet* (Anonymous, 1985). The editorial reported the results of the Belgian study and called for an RCT to evaluate the relationship between episiotomy and third-degree tears. Interest in the issue continued with letters to the editor of the *British Journal of Obstetrics and Gynaecology* (Blondel & Kaminski, 1985) and the *Lancet* (Dunn, 1985; Buekens *et al.*, 1986).

It was also in 1985 that the European and American regional offices of the World Health Organization and the Pan American Health Organization held a conference on appropriate technology for birth. The delegates to the conference accepted childbirth as a natural and normal process. Among the list of recommendations unanimously adopted by the conference was one rejecting the routine use of episiotomy.

'The perineum should be protected wherever possible. Systematic use of episiotomy is not justified' (World Health Organization, 1985:437).

Although published in the *Lancet* and later in the *AIMS Quarterly Journal* (Beech, 1987a), these recommendations appear not to have been widely disseminated in the UK. Two years earlier, the lack of evidence for the routine use of episiotomy was also published in the English language journal of the Scandinavian Association of Obstetricians and Gynecologists, *Acta Obstetricia et Gynecologica Scandinavica*. This paper, which was written in preparation for the 1985 conference, reviewed the literature for the scientific basis for use and the psycho-social effects of perinatal procedures (Fraser, 1983).

Strategies for bringing about change

During the 1970s in the UK, the rationales for routine episiotomy were largely taken for granted. An examination of the professional literature critical of routine episiotomy reveals three ways in which opponents went about undermining these rationales. First, similar to American physicians who advocated routine episiotomy based on clinical assumptions rather than empirical evidence, some of the earliest episiotomy critiques relied heavily on clinical experience and common-sense to argue against the practice (e.g. Levett, 1974; Willmott, 1979; 1980). The following passage from Willmott is typical of this sort of argument.

'The advocates of such policies [routine episiotomy] suggest that women have an inbuilt pelvic "flaw". A lot of irresponsible medical propaganda is being put about claiming that unless an episiotomy is performed there will be stretching and damage of the pelvic supports, leading to prolapse in later life. If they were correct, it would seem strange that evolution should have produced such an imperfect structure, wouldn't it?' (Willmott, 1981:26)

As suggested by the quotation, this type of critique questions the need for episiotomy by challenging the existing obstetric belief system supporting the practice. These critics refuted the argument that the functioning of the perineum during childbirth was pathological (i.e. produced prolapse in later life). By invoking the philosophical argument that childbirth was actually a normal process, they held that routine surgical intervention was not required. As the following passage reveals, this type of reasoning is remarkably similar to the one made by late nineteenth-century physicians who resisted the pleas for the more liberal use of episiotomy. Pondering a remark made by an eminent American physician that lacerations of the uterus were quite common, Samuel Gross, Emeritus Professor of Surgery at Jefferson Medical College, Philadelphia and founder of the American Surgical Association, commented in 1884:

'If it be true, it would inevitably go to prove that God has made woman much less perfect than the world has given him credit for. As childbirth is one of the special perogatives of women, designed to perpetuate the race, there is something peculiarly distressing in such an idea. Looking at the matter from a practical standpoint, one would naturally conclude that the Author of our being had constructed the womb with special care to protect the organ, at least as a rule, against the possibility of contingency fraught with such sad consequences. If we assume the correctness of Dr Emmet's statement, we may well wonder, without irreverence, why Almighty God did not create simultaneously with woman a competent gynecologist, ready to meet this inevitable evil, for which such unquestionably it must be whenever it occurs' (Gross, 1884; 338).

Other examples of this type of questioning appear in leading articles, editorials and letters to the editor of various journals pointing out the lack of research supporting the routine use of episiotomy and calling for the practice to be re-evaluated scientifically (e.g. Anonymous, 1968; Zander, 1982). These challenges, which were largely non-evidence-based in the sense that they did not present the results of studies conducted by the authors, raised consciousness of the operation by sensitizing the average clinician to the fact that there was growing disagreement within professional circles about the value of the practice. In some cases, these presentations also had the effect of provoking clinicians who strongly believed in the practice to come to its defence (e.g. Flood, 1982). This helped to further bring the episiotomy debate out into the open and create greater uncertainty about the claims which had been made for performing the operation.

A second and more convincing type of critique relies on reviews of the literature to challenge the very basis on which the practice of episiotomy had been built, that is, the benefits claimed for the procedure. These papers, more difficult for clinicians to dismiss outright than the non-evidence-based criticisms, produced greater uncertainty about the value of episiotomy. They did so by revealing that little evidence existed in the literature supporting the rationales which had been offered for the operation. House's 1981 review is an example of this type of critique:

'...but it must be stressed at the outset that there is an almost complete lack of any scientific evidence that the operation has any of the beneficial effects claimed for it. A search of the literature has failed to reveal any study designed to compare the effects on mother and baby of doing or not doing episiotomies...It would be expected that for a standard procedure that is performed hundreds of thousands of times every year there would be solid evidence in the world literature comparing the results of delivery without episiotomy. Without such evidence, how could such a widespread procedure become so well established? In fact, no such evidence exists' (House, 1981a:6,8).

The third type of critique, and the one probably thought to be the most influential in bringing about change in medicine, challenges the alleged benefits of routine episiotomy with actual data from recently conducted research. These studies, which included observational studies (e.g. Needham & Sheriff, 1983; Wilkerson, 1984; Gordon & Logue, 1985) as well as prospective RCTs (Harrison *et al.*, 1984; Sleep *et al.*, 1984; House *et al.*, 1986), set out to evaluate the claims made about episiotomy, but were typically unable to produce evidence supporting routine use of the procedure.

The effect of questioning

Unfortunately national data for England on episiotomy rates for 1979 and 1981–1984 are unavailable. This makes it impossible to establish exactly when episiotomy rates began falling or how the rate of decline in the use of episiotomy changed during these years. Data does exist for one hospital for the period 1980–1984 (Reynolds & Yudkin, 1987). In the four years between 1980 and 1984, the episiotomy rate at the Oxford Radcliffe NHS Trust Hospital declined by 27.7% in absolute terms for primips and 21.4% for multips (Fig. 5). This represents a relative rate of decline in episiotomy use of 38.2% for primips and 58.2% for multips. When the relative rate of change is calculated for individual years, the greatest reductions occurred between 1983 and 1984 (17.8%) and 1981 and 1982 (16%) for primips. For multips, the greatest declines also occurred between 1983 and 1984 (27.7%) and 1981 and 1982 (26.5%).

It should be noted that the decline in episiotomy at Oxford Radcliffe Hospital cannot be explained away by changes in other obstetric interventions which also may have been occurring at the same time.

> '...since the fall in the episiotomy rate was the most striking of all the changes [obstetric interventions], it seems to have had its own momentum and not to have been dependent on other changes in the management of the second stage (Reynolds & Yudkin, 1987:1048).

When these data are juxtaposed with the questioning of episiotomy which was taking place between 1980 and 1984, it appears that the non-evidence-based episiotomy critiques, which began accumulating in a significant way only in 1982, had an impact on the use of the operation.

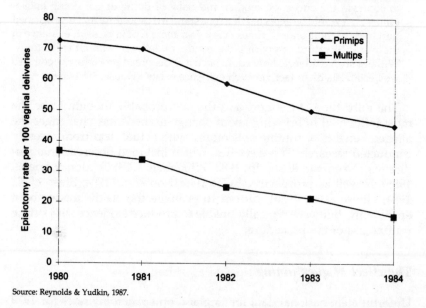

Source: Reynolds & Yudkin, 1987.

Fig. 5   Episiotomy rate for Oxford Radcliffe NHS Trust Hospital (1980–1984).

The evidence-based critiques on the other hand, played little role in bringing about the initial reduction in the use of the operation. While the vast majority of evidence-based critiques did not appear in print until the late summer and autumn of 1984, the episiotomy rate had already dropped in absolute terms – 22.8% for primips and 15.5% for multips – by 1983.

Unfortunately, the Reynolds and Yudkin study examines the episiotomy rate only up to 1984, the year the results of two of the RCTs were published. This makes it impossible to know the extent to which the results of these trials may have further stimulated a decline in the use of episiotomy. Unlike the 1982 editorial in the *BMJ* by Russell (Russell, 1982) which stimulated the medical debate about the use of episiotomy, neither the Dublin nor West Berkshire RCTs generated much discussion in the literature. In all, both trials prompted only three letters to the editor. One letter related to the 'informed consent' procedures followed in the Dublin study (Neville-Smith, 1984); another by a biomathematician challenged the interpretation of the results of the Dublin study on methodological grounds (Läärä, 1984); and the third wished for a more definitive statement from the West Berkshire trial that episiotomy is not beneficial and should not be carried out (Lewis, 1984).

While it is not possible to quantify the effect these two RCTs may have had on clinicians' use of episiotomy, they had an impact in the literature. The results of these trials were cited by clinicians and childbirth advocates to justify abandoning the routine use of episiotomy (Kitzinger, 1984; Sleep *et al.*, 1989). While the results of the RCTs may not have produced the initial reduction in the use of episiotomy, these trials were nonetheless extremely important because they provided for the first time a scientific rationale for the limited use of episiotomy, which had already come about.

Obstetrical and midwifery interest in questioning episiotomy

Having traced the development of professional criticism of routine episiotomy and discussed its relationship with the use of the operation, it is also useful to consider some of the factors that motivated this questioning. The critiques themselves and interviews with the key informants offer insights into what some of these factors might have been.

Midwifery interest in questioning episiotomy

Midwifery interest in questioning episiotomy and midwives' receptivity to such questioning were very much related to the issue of professional preservation; both in terms of maintaining a particular skill (management of the perineum) and in terms of the broader concept of professional autonomy. For many of the midwives who authored episiotomy critiques, the trend toward the routine use of episiotomy was perceived to be a serious threat to the traditional and revered midwifery skill of managing the perineum so as to minimize perineal trauma. Delivery over an intact perineum was and is considered one of the hallmarks of midwifery skill. Midwives were concerned that as more and more of their cohort and midwives in training cut episiotomies, the skill of managing the perineum with the intention of leaving the perineum intact would be lost.

> 'Through psychoprophylaxis, we are helping our mothers to be controlled with their pushing, to co-operate with the midwife by resisting the pushing urge at crowning. Are not these skills and the potential skills of the midwife being thwarted by the increasing frequency of episiotomy?' (Levett, 1974)

> 'It was always considered, in the past, that the supreme skill of the midwife was her ability, in most cases, gently to deliver the baby, leaving the mother unscathed, with an intact perineum... It is a matter of judgment... Surely it all boils down to good midwifery. Mechanical practices, like routine episiotomy, are tending to mar the beauty of childbirth' (Willmott, 1979).

> 'The midwifery skill of perineal management is under threat of extinction; this has been brought about largely as a consequence of reduced professional confidence, coupled with a growing obsession with the role of episiotomy to the exclusion of other aspects of perineal management during and following childbirth' (Sleep, 1987:455).

The questioning of episiotomy also had to do with asserting midwives' professional autonomy by resisting an intervention they perceived as being imposed by obstetricians. As described in Chapter 4, the routine use of episiotomy was in part related to the increasing involvement of medical practitioners in normal maternity care as childbirth moved from home to hospital. Episiotomy was one of many obstetrical practices that midwives were encouraged (or even ordered) by obstetricians to take up. For many midwives, this came to symbolize the medical take-over of midwifery decision-making in the management of normal labour. As one midwife has observed:

> 'The end of the 1970s was in many ways a turning-point for the profession, with the recognition that certain trends in the health services over the past two decades had undermined various aspects of their contribution to maternity care' (Robinson, 1990:81).

Mary Renfrew, author (Renfrew *et al.*, 1990; Enkin *et al.*, 1995) and Professor of Midwifery at the University of Leeds, has described what happened in the following way:

'from the 1960s through into the 1970s there was an increase in routine intervention that midwives simply took on board for a while, although there were movements against it, but for a while, it swept over the midwifery profession very fast. And *then* all of a sudden people started to say that, "This isn't right because we never used to do that and it was never a problem before". And they would target single practices ... And episiotomy was one of the big ones because of course lots of midwives didn't want to do routine episiotomy, had never done them before so why should they now? And the younger ones started to say, "Well how do I deliver babies without episiotomy? You know, teach me". So as the move against episiotomy started to happen, as I understand it from my own personal experience from the late 1970s, 1979 through 1984 probably was a very important period for midwives turning against episiotomy. It may have been happening earlier than that, but I was not aware of it.

Then midwives started to say, we don't have to do this stuff. They were also starting to say, we don't have to do routine monitoring, we don't have to do certain things ... position in labour was another one. Why were women all lying down these days in labour, why aren't they up and about? And, if you like, that was a return to midwifery practice as it used to occur, but for a while got swept over with the move into hospital. Then they started to say, "Hey, we have to stop doing that"' (interview with Mary Renfrew).

In publicly questioning episiotomy, midwives were resisting obstetrical intrusion into midwifery decision-making and reasserting their professional independence. These critiques were intended to draw attention to the fact that by performing episiotomy routinely, midwives were surrendering 'yet one more area of their specialist professional knowledge to the obstetrician' (Kitzinger, 1979a:233). The following passage from Sleep offers a sense of the strong desire some midwives felt about the need for the midwifery profession to be self-directing and midwives to regain the freedom to exercise clinical judgement.

'And the way that it [Kitzinger and Walter's *Some Women's Experiences of Episiotomy* 1981) lent impetus to what I was doing was her concluding sentence which was, "It is up to obstetricians who perform this invasive procedure to justify that its benefits outweigh its hazards". And I think that is verbatim. Because I had thought, it is not obstetricians who do episiotomies, it is midwives. In 75% of vaginal deliveries, the senior person present is the midwife. Midwives do episiotomies not obstetricians. And I thought, well if we don't look at it, an obstetrician will and will turn around and make recommendations to the midwifery practice. And we have really got to stand up and do something about it' (interview with Jennifer Sleep).

Medical interest in questioning episiotomy

The reasons for medical interest in questioning episiotomy are much less clear. Some physicians, like Iain Chalmers (author of a 1976 episiotomy critique, former Director of the National Perinatal Epide-miology Unit, co-investigator of the West Berkshire episiotomy RCT) and Michael House (author of several episiotomy critiques and prin-cipal investigator of the London RCT), raised questions about routine episiotomy out of strong personal convictions that obstetric practice should be based on evidence rather than the opinion of authorities. It is interesting to note that both men believe they were greatly influenced by practising obstetrics in developing countries early in their careers. During these periods, they found that much of what they had been taught in medical school about the need for obstetrical intervention in childbirth did not apply to the women they were assisting to deliver. These observations raised doubts in their minds about the evidence for obstetrical interventions.

'The thing that changed my *life* was working in a Palestinian refugee camp for two years. *There* I saw women having babies without any sort of inter-vention, many having reasonably good outcome of pregnancy, and it raised in my mind the question of what is the evidence to justify all the things that are done in my home country. So it was the experience of working with the Palestinians that made me question the need for many of the things that were being done in my own community back home. *That's* what did it, and it wasn't specifically with episiotomy although episiotomy was extremely rare there. I don't know, but the fact of the matter was, that stitching after childbirth was actually quite rarely needed in that particular community. And episiotomy was done exceedingly ... very, very, very rarely indeed. So, that was just part of a general sort of *up-ending* of so many assumptions that I had' (interview with Iain Chalmers).

'I trained in this country and then a year after qualification I went to the West Indies on a two year contract and stayed there ten years. Now, over there, where I was anyhow, it was on a small island, there weren't many midwives and more or less no doctors. So episiotomy was very rarely performed. And a lot of patients had a large number of children and, from my observation, perineal lacerations were not a big problem. They didn't seem to be any more common than I remembered them here. And long-term problems of perineal discomfort or prolapse or whatever else you talk about didn't seem to be bad. So when I came back to this country, and came to this unit, I found that even though this unit prided itself on ... a non-interventionalist sort of natural approach to obstetrics, that the episiotomy rate in primigravids anyhow was extraordinarily high. I mean it was nearly 80% in primigravids. And ... it was so high that it was almost the policy to, not quite but almost the policy to, do episiotomy in most people having their first baby, unless they strongly objected for some reason. And I thought this was a bad policy...' (interview with Michael House).

Something else that was extremely important, if not crucial, in prompting the production of many of the professional episiotomy critiques was pressure from outside the professions to re-evaluate the practice. This pressure came largely from Sheila Kitzinger, the NCT, the AIMS and ultimately childbearing women.

Women initiating and nurturing professional controversy

By 1972, when the episiotomy rate had risen appreciably, Sheila Kitzinger, perhaps the most influential authority on childbirth education, was the first to raise serious concerns about its routine use. Kitzinger, prompted by 'the large number of accounts of painful stitching and postpartum discomfort which arrived on the National Childbirth Trust headquarters' desk' (Kitzinger, 1972:preface), edited a booklet on episiotomy for the NCT entitled *Episiotomy. Physical and Emotional Aspects.* The NCT is *the* organization in the UK devoted to childbirth education. It is a large organization with 40 000 members and includes antenatal teachers (know as prenatal or childbirth educators in the USA and Canada), parents and midwives (Kitzinger, 1990:92).

Kitzinger's booklet, intended for those working in midwifery, obstetrics and antenatal teaching, suggested ways to reduce episiotomy and presented technical advice on means of reducing complications when episiotomy was necessary. In retrospect, this document launched a lay campaign to reduce the indiscriminate use of episiotomy. By reporting women's negative experiences of the operation, Kitzinger essentially legitimatized and validated these women's experiences.

Furthermore, based on a small survey of 145 NCT women's experiences with episiotomy, Kitzinger suggested that the iatrogenic episiotomy complications, which had up until this time been considered only a problem experienced by a few individual women, might actually be much more widespread. The survey revealed that a sizeable proportion of respondents complained of pain at the time their episiotomy incision was stitched. The other issue the survey identified as a problem was the amount of time some women were waiting to have their episiotomy wound sutured.

In the years to follow, public awareness of the operation was heightened by articles in the popular British press which reported on the devastating emotional and sexual side-effects of the operation and called for a reappraisal of the whole subject of episiotomy. One of the earliest was Froshaug's (1974) 'The unkindest cut of all?' published in *Nova*, a 'glossy "socially aware" women's magazine' (Kitzinger, 1990:96). This article, published a month before the appearance of the first midwifery critique, focused attention on the impact of a 'clumsy incision and incorrect stitching' on women's future health, both physically and sexually, by telling several women's terrible experiences with the operation.

During the mid 1970s, the lay questioning of episiotomy intensified when the AIMS began publicizing women's dissatisfaction with episiotomy and overtly campaigning against the operation. AIMS is a national maternity care pressure group which has been at the forefront of questioning maternity practices in the UK since 1960.

AIMS' opposition to routine episiotomy developed as women suffering from the most serious and unpleasant episiotomy complications began contacting the organization seeking its help and advice. Using the *AIMS Quarterly Newsletter* as a campaigning document, AIMS illustrated the devastating effects the operation could have on the birth experience as well as women's lives, questioned the routine use of episiotomy, demanded that fewer episiotomies be performed and insisted that those that were performed be done with greater care.

In March 1976, the *AIMS Quarterly Newsletter* began publicizing women's complaints about episiotomy. An article by an anonymous contributor expressed AIMS' anger concerning problems related to repair of the incision (Anonymous, 1976). The following passages provide an indication of the tone of the article and the impact that episiotomy problems had on some women.

'It is therefore of great concern that stitching should be conducted by highly skilled personnel. Often episiotomies are left to medical students for practice. Young men who have never held a needle and thread before learn their first surgical skills on this most precious part of the female anatomy. When complaints are made by mothers of pain months later (and strained marital relations), these are dismissed as meuroses [sic]. Tranquillizers are administered – which may cure a sore mind, but hardly a sore seat!'

'Another source of complaint is the way doctors treat mothers after episiotomy. In the majority of cases, midwives deliver the baby, then leave the delivery room. The mother then waits (often hours) for a (usually strange) doctor to stitch the wound. Not only can this be extremely humiliating for the mother, but it must also be the least rewarding part of obstetrics to the doctor. He or she has not shared in the birth experience, and therefore has no involvement with the mother. Thus the natural exhilaration felt by the mother after the birth of her baby is squashed by complete lack of sympathy' (Anonymous, 1976).

Also in March, members of AIMS met with officials of the Maternity Services Department of the Department of Health and Social Services (DHSS) to raise maternity care issues of concern to AIMS. The problem of bad episiotomy repairs was brought up by the AIMS delegates. They informed the Department officials that AIMS was disconcerted to learn that medical students at one prestigious London medical school were carrying out episiotomies and repairing them despite never before having done any stitching on anyone (AIMS Quarterly Newsletter, 1976:9). The Department officials appeared not to take this concern seriously as they replied by saying, 'Well, they have to learn on someone'.

In October 1977, the *AIMS Quarterly Newsletter* featured a second and more informative piece on episiotomy (Pallet, 1977). Previously, AIMS had requested women's experiences with episiotomy in *Mother and Baby* magazine and received responses from 13 mothers. The article summarized and presented these mothers' horrendous experiences, often quoting them directly. This article concluded by attempting to provoke professionals to do something about women's complaints concerning episiotomy.

> 'The NCT published a booklet "Episiotomy. Physical and Emotional Aspects", written by sympathetic professionals (midwives, doctors, etc.) which makes many of the same points as these letters. It was written five years ago and the letters we have received this year are making the same complaints. Perhaps we need some research into episiotomy and its consequences, if only to prevent the sort of unnecessary suffering that goes on, more important in a way, to avoid endangering or jeopardizing vital relationships such as that between a woman and her husband, and a mother and her child' (Pallet, 1977:4).

By the end of 1978, the NCT renewed its interest in episiotomy when it again started asking if routine episiotomy was really necessary. This questioning was picked up and repeated in the popular press as indicated by an article in the *The Guardian* (Adamson, 1978).

By the spring of 1979, when the routine use of episiotomy was just beginning to be questioned in the midwifery literature, lay questioning of the practice had already reached substantial proportions. For example, Willmott in her 1979 midwifery critique acknowledges the 'rising tide of professional and lay opinion against this wholesale practice [routine episiotomy]'. Some obstetricians were also beginning to feel the heat of women's questioning of the procedure. For example, in a 1979 paper explaining how to perform and repair episiotomy incision, J.S. Fox, Senior Lecturer in Obstetrics at Charing Cross Hospital Medical School in London remarked that episiotomy:

> '... is often under fire from our militant "consumers" who maintain that episiotomies are often done unnecessarily and that the pain subsequently experienced in the puerperium from this "unkindest cut of all" interferes with bonding between mother and baby' (Fox, 1979:337).

At exactly this same time Kitzinger (1979a), frustrated by the midwifery profession's apparent willingness to accept and even perform routine episiotomy, brought the episiotomy debate directly to the attention of midwives by writing a critique on episiotomy which was published in one of the profession's own journals. In the 'controversy' section of the widely read *Midwife, Health Visitor and Community Nurse*, Kitzinger discussed the iatrogenic complications produced by episiotomy, disputed the claim that episiotomy prevented subsequent gynaecological problems and appealed to midwives to reject routine episiotomy in favour of their traditional skill of delivering women with minimal perineal trauma.

In 1979, Kitzinger also published *The Good Birth Guide* (1979b). In this bestseller, she summarized reports she received from a total of 1800 women with experiences in maternity units from across the country and issued stars for each maternity unit's sensitivity to women's childbearing needs. While the focus of the book was on the treatment of childbearing women in maternity units, the issue of episiotomy figured prominently throughout. For example, when Kitzinger's informers included information on a unit's use of episiotomy, this information was included in the *Guide*, as was any information provided by the units themselves. Episiotomy was also discussed in a section of the book explaining obstetrical procedures commonly encountered during childbirth. Kitzinger challenged the practice of routine episiotomy and urged expectant mothers to discuss all aspects of episiotomy with their caregivers in advance. She also encouraged them to tell their attendants if they wanted to be helped to manage their birth without an episiotomy.

This book had a phenomenal impact on professionals. For the first time, many of them were made aware that they provided a service and that consumers had preferences which they considered important and wished to have respected. Furthermore, anecdotal evidence suggests this book 'prompted some British maternity units to abandon some routine practices unsupported by any good evidence' (Banta, 1989:1455). This interpretation is also supported by such diverse and prominent individuals as Chalmers (1975; 1976a;b; *et al.*, 1989), Zander (1982), Flint (1985; 1986) and Beech (1987a;b; 1991; 1996).

'Oh, I think, if I was to identify one single thing which had opened up the debate about childbirth in this country it would be Sheila Kitzinger's *The Good Birth Guide*. I think she probably did more to ... push proper consideration of women's needs in childbirth into a forum for debate by publication of that book that any other single person has done with any other intervention they have made in this whole area. So far as I am concerned she is a big heroine for having published that book. It gave maternity hospitals evidence that they had a public face and that this was published for people to see' (interview with Iain Chalmers).

'... she wrote *The Good Birth Guide* rather like a WHICH? report [a monthly consumer magazine which carries out surveys of the quality of consumer goods] or a good food guide or something, and people were furious – obstetricians. Absolutely furious. "How unmethodical. What sort of a report is this? How can you judge quality by one person?" Because what she did was just ask for comments from mothers. And sometimes there was only one comment from one mother from a hospital or two comments or three or whatever ... It's very anecdotal but ... it had an effect. And I think it had an effect by again demonstrating something which is more advanced in America, the realization of the importance of the consumer view. But I think that in maternity care, people began to realize that the consumer view had a potential for changing things' (interview with Luke Zander).

'Yes, yes. Sheila Kitzinger has been a very ... well, she has just changed so much. I mean, one of the most dramatic things that she has ever done was doing *The Good Birth Guide*. I mean, the anger it engendered. And she did all the, you know, these stars for maternity units. Maternity units were *incensed*. "What was this woman doing? She wasn't even a midwife, she wasn't even a doctor and she was saying, she was questioning our practice. Huh!" And they were so angry. And you see, she, I think for the first time, she pointed out to midwives and doctors, she said, "You're providing us with a service, the service you are providing is not pleasing us. Get your finger out"' (interview with Caroline Flint).

'And *The Good Birth Guide* had an influence, most certainly had an influence because she was the one who ... she had obstetricians ringing her up when they had only got one star saying, "We have changed a lot of things and we are doing this and you know ... it is much better now, much better now. We've had a total change of staff". And terribly keen to make sure they got into the next one, you know, got into the next publication so that their hospital got four or five stars. *The Good Birth Guide* was very useful in focusing attention on choice and making them realize that women actually had the choice to do that and to move around' (interview with Beverley Lawrence Beech).

The momentum for questioning maternity practices generated by the *The Good Birth Guide* was maintained by the release of *The New Good Birth Guide* in 1983 which was a revision and update of the earlier book.

Also in 1979, the NCT and AIMS joined forces to raise professional awareness of lay opposition to routine episiotomy. The two childbirth organizations jointly approached the national British DHSS to criticize the indiscriminate use of episiotomy. Complaining to the DHSS about the rate of episiotomy succeeded in getting the government department to publicly state its opposition to the routine use of the operation. The DHSS replied to AIMS and the NCT by saying:

'We would never be happy to see a procedure such as episiotomy regarded as "routine". Our policy has been and will continue to be that the needs of the individual patient are paramount. We regard as unacceptable the setting of any arbitrary time limit in the second stage of labour, after which episiotomy or forceps delivery would automatically be performed without regard to the clinical circumstances' (Anonymous, 1979).

Two other influential activities that Kitzinger and the NCT undertook specifically related to the issue of episiotomy also began in early 1979. Between March 1979 and 1980, Kitzinger and Walters, in colla- boration with the NCT, conducted a survey of 1795 NCT mothers' subjective experiences with episiotomy and the subsequent suturing. In September 1981, the NCT published the results of Kitzinger's epi siotomy study under the title *Some Women's Experiences of Episiotomy* (Kitzinger & Walters, 1981). The most striking findings of the survey were that women who had had episiotomies:

- experienced more pain at the end of the first week postpartum than women who had lacerations;
- found it more difficult to get into or maintain a comfortable position to breastfeed than women with lacerations;
- were more likely to experience dyspareunia (painful intercourse) and for a longer period than those with lacerations.

Pain during suturing and waiting to be sutured also appeared as common problems experienced by women.

Having documented that women receiving an episiotomy (as opposed to remaining intact or experiencing a spontaneous second- degree tear) experienced greater pain and dyspareunia, Kitzinger and Walters concluded their report by challenging physicians to either prove the benefits of episiotomy or stop performing it.

> 'Episiotomy causes women often unnecessary pain at and following delivery. It does not, despite claims to the contrary, avoid tears, does not improve the condition of the perineum in the weeks following childbirth, may interfere with the mother's initial relationship with her baby and the start of breastfeeding and can adversely affect the couple's sexual relation- ship for a long time after.'

> 'It is up to women to refuse to give consent to any intervention unless it can be shown to be necessary and evidence is produced to back up this claim. It is up to obstetricians who make this surgical wound to prove that its benefits outweigh its hazards, or to stop a practice which is demonstrably harmful to many women and causes a great deal of needless suffering' (Kitzinger & Walters, 1981:10).

At the same time as *Some Women's Experiences of Episiotomy* was released, the NCT also released an updated and expanded version of Kitzinger's 1972 booklet *Episiotomy. Physical and Emotional Aspects* (Kitzinger, 1981). In this version, all but Kitzinger's chapter was written by health care professionals sympathetic to women's concerns about the overuse of episiotomy (House, 1981b; Willmott, 1981). Two of the chapters were reprints or modified versions of earlier articles; Will- mott's 1980 critique which appeared in *Midwives Chronicle and Nursing*

Notes, and House's 1981 episiotomy literature review which appeared in *Midwife, Health Visitor and Community Nurse* (1981a). Both NCT publications were extremely critical of the operation and called for a reduction in its use.

Not surprisingly given Kitzinger's stature and media connections, the results of her episiotomy survey were widely reported in both *The Sunday Times* (Gillie, 1981) and *The Times* (of London) (Haigh, 1981), newspapers with circulations of several million. Two weeks before the booklets were released by the NCT, Walters, Kitzinger's research assistant and co-author on the episiotomy survey, further publicized the lay questioning of episiotomy by drawing midwives' attention to the fact that physicians seemed completely disinterested in questioning the practice despite women's concern about the issue. In a one page article in *Nursing Times*, Walters noted:

'...it is distressing to find while women are questioning the practice of episiotomy, while it has well documented risks, and while none of the benefits claimed for it are adequately demonstrated, none of this concern is reflected in the medical journals. Obstetricians are debating about whether to perform midline or mediolateral episiotomy, and whether to stitch with catgut or polyglycolic acid, while many mothers and midwives are finding that their rather different priorities are ignored or dismissed' (1981:14).

There can be little doubt that Kitzinger's episiotomy booklets and all the attention they received in the media had a considerable impact. As the following passages reveal, Kitzinger's episiotomy activities were in large part responsible for provoking Russell's 1982 *BMJ* editorial and the episiotomy debate that subsequently ensued in the correspondence section of this journal. Russell's editorial was published almost six months to the day after the release of Kitzinger's booklets.

'With increasing insistence individual women, and sometimes well-organized groups, are asking whether some procedure is manifestly to the advantage of mother and baby or amounts to unnecessary interference by doctors... The spotlight of public concern has now moved to episiotomy. The National Childbirth Trust has recently published a collection of essays on the physical and emotional aspects of episiotomy with contributions from obstetricians and midwives, concluding with Sheila Kitzinger's assessment of its effects on postnatal adjustment... All these studies show how many questions remain unanswered' (Russell, 1982).

It is not until the last paragraph of the editorial, however, that the success women were having in challenging episiotomy becomes clear.

'...And as women become better informed and more articulate they are sure to have strong views on this important subject. It would, however, be a pity if clinical practice were changed on insufficient evidence of a patient-led protest. The answers should come from clinical research' (Russell, 1982).

Not only were Kitzinger and her activities instrumental in prompting the Russell editorial, she also entered the medical debate by writing a letter to the editor of the *BMJ* in response to the editorial. In her letter, she reviewed the results of her episiotomy study and ended it by chastising physicians for not taking it upon themselves to question the practice.

'The onus is on obstetricians to justify intervention, of whatever kind, not on women to prove that it is harmful. With episiotomy, as with induction, it should be a matter of some concern that criticism has had to come from outside the profession before obstetricians themselves got down to questioning a routine practice' (Kitzinger, 1982).

The lay questioning of childbirth practices became even more difficult for professionals to ignore with the founding of the Active Childbirth Movement in April 1982. This movement developed in response to the action of a London hospital in banning 'Active Birth'. 'Active Birth' is the term used by women wanting to give birth in upright positions (Balaskas, 1989:x). To protest the hospital's policy which denied women the freedom to move around in labour and assume any birthing position they chose, Janet Balaskas, who developed the concept of Active Birth, organized a Birthrights Rally with AIMS and the Birth Centre Movement members. The rally drew a crowd of 6000 to the hospital on a Sunday afternoon. Sheila Kitzinger and Michael Odent, a French obstetrician, were speakers at the rally. Following the demonstration, the physician responsible for the decision to ban Active Birth resigned as Professor and women wanting Active Births were accommodated by the hospital.

A survey conducted by a television programme generated additional discussion about childbirth practices that same year. The programme received nearly 10 000 letters and nearly 6000 women returned questionnaires (Jacoby & Cartwright, 1990:250). The results of the survey were later published as *The British Way of Birth* (Boyd & Sellers, 1982). Regarding episiotomy, the survey revealed three issues of concern to women.

'The strongest comments on episiotomies and tears came firstly from women who had to wait a long time for a doctor to come and put stitches in – sometimes for several hours – when the stitches were frequently painful and in some cases more painful than the delivery. Secondly, many women mentioned with great gratitude midwives who helped them to give birth in such a way as to avoid the need for an episiotomy or a tear – by slow and gentle stretching. Other women said they wished they had been cut rather than torn' (Boyd & Sellers, 1982:120).

While generally refraining from questioning the benefits of the liberal use of episiotomy, Boyd and Sellers did conclude their discussion of episiotomy by expressing concern that when episiotomy is performed routinely, the midwifery skill of guarding the perineum is lost.

This television programme and the subsequent book did much to heighten the public's awareness of maternity practices including episiotomy. As Chalmers notes:

'*The British Way of Birth* ... was a big survey done through a television programme, consumer orientated television programme, called "That's Life", which was introduced by a woman called Esther Rantzen. And that was extremely influential in raising people's awareness of what was going on. That was published as a paperback, *The British Way of Birth*. You know, inductions, episiotomy, Caesarean sections, position during birth, all of those things got raised in that. So there has been a very, very vibrant debate going on in this country about childbirth, no shadow of a doubt about that. And I don't know that it has gone on in quite the same way in other European countries' (interview with Iain Chalmers).

Another event took place in 1982 which further helped bolster lay opposition to traditional obstetrical management of childbirth. That year, Sally Inch's book *Birthrights. What Every Parent Should Know About Childbirth in Hospitals* became a bestseller in the UK. In the book, Inch, a community midwife in Oxford, described all of the obstetrical practices commonly performed during childbirth and carefully assessed the evidence for each one. Specifically regarding episiotomy, Inch devoted a total of 16 pages to the practice. She presented each of the rationales offered by physicians for performing the operation and then methodically disputed each one.

Beverley Lawrence Beech, the Honorary chair of AIMS, describes yet one other lay activity that occurred in 1982 which contributed to changing the midwifery profession's view of routine episiotomy.

'I mean, routine episiotomy was something we were constantly *screaming* about. You see, in 1982 we launched the Maternity Defence Fund, that was the most significant thing we did. The Maternity Defence Fund ... we were so fed up with women coming to us and saying, "I didn't want this drip [IV], I didn't want pethidine [demeral], I didn't want an episiotomy'. Pethidine was one of the major things that ... they were told ... you know, you are so many centimetres – pethidine. And the women would say, "I'd rather you didn't do that. I don't want that". "Oh, it's our policy." And there was no argument, they got it. The same thing happened with episiotomy. Women would say, "I'd rather not have one" and they would be told, 'It's our policy". So we said, "Right. We are going to sue you for assault. We've had enough". And within weeks the medical press, the midwifery press, were full of articles discussing informed consent. They had never discussed it up till then seriously, there had been nothing serious about informed consent.

Suddenly we have discussions about informed consent' (interview with Beverley Lawrence Beech).

As Beech claims, the Maternity Defence Fund (MDF) did stimulate professional interest in re-evaluating the routine use of episiotomy. For example, within two weeks of the press release announcing the launch of the MDF, two articles appeared in *Nursing Mirror* dealing with the issue. One was by a patient activist explaining the reasons why patients were going to sue professionals (Robinson, 1982), and the other by a barrister, explaining the legal ramifications of informed consent (Finch, 1982). The following passages from the barrister's article must have encouraged some midwives to rethink the meaning of informed consent, as well as the routine use of episiotomy.

'The law says, in clear and unambiguous terms, that an unwarranted interference with another person's body without that person's consent, or the lawful consent of a person recognized as entitled to give that consent, is an assault. Or rather, to be strictly legally accurate, a battery.... A "routine" (unnecessary or objected to) episiotomy is a serious assault (and battery) against a patient. It is no different in law from a knife wound delivered in a fight' (Finch, 1982).

Further evidence that lay questioning of episiotomy stimulated professional questioning of the practice as well as encouraged the declining use of the operation comes from several sources. Chalmers describes the events that led to the midwifery questioning of episiotomy in the following way:

'Women themselves start it off. Midwives came into the debate, but it was women who started the whole thing rolling. And they used whatever evidence they could and whatever support they could from professionals who joined in. Midwives came in, I would say, very late in the day, they were brought along by women. Obviously, some of the midwives most active in those debates were, indeed, not just young midwives who wanted to sort of challenge the status quo, but also midwives who had had babies themselves and who had felt fed up with some of the things that went on when they were having babies. So I'd say that midwives started to come in about 1979, but that was sort of seven or eight years after women had started this whole thing going. So, I think this is a very encouraging example of consumer power actually creating a debate, the extent to which they have been able to actually change the system is another question. But in terms of the credit for actually getting the debate going, it's theirs' (interview with Iain Chalmers).

Luke Zander, author of the editorial 'Episiotomy: has familiarity bred contempt?', also identifies Kitzinger as the driving force behind much of the flurry of professional interest in episiotomy which took place in the 1980s, particularly around 1982. Responding to a question about what had led to so much medical and midwifery interest in episiotomy in the early 1980s, Zander replied:

'Sheila Kitzinger! She had an enormous effect... My own reading of what's happened is that if you do something which runs counter or discredits a procedure, it is exceedingly difficult to get this from within. And in issues of birth I think there are a number of examples where the community-based studies and pressure have had amazing effect. Now, episiotomy is one because Sheila did this study of her 2000 NCT mothers. Now that was the first time, as far as I remember, that there had been any serious look at what were the benefits or otherwise of episiotomies, *anywhere* in the Western literature. And that was in 1981. And it caused a great deal of ... it got a great deal of publicity. There were a few people who were very struck by Sheila's approach or report, it played a big part in making people have to rethink the issue. It took an issue which hadn't been done before and then ... I mean, everyone said, "Why it's not scientific, they just asked NCT people". But it was the first time in the literature, as far as I remember, that anyone questioned whether this was really necessary ... this was a figure of 2000 women. So then a few people sat down and started doing some medical, obstetric research. But ... the initial stimulus came from pressure from outside the profession' (interview with Luke Zander).

From a midwifery perspective, Sleep also identifies Kitzinger and her NCT booklets as agents of change.

'Well of course that was when Sheila published her *Some Women's Experiences*, which I'm sure was instrumental in spearheading the whole thing. And Sheila's purple booklet was launched and the whole paperback was launched in quite a big blaze of publicity because she mobilizes a powerful machinery when she publishes. So it had a huge press coverage in the national media and so it was hard to ignore. I mean, whether you were a woman or a professional, she was highlighting the lack of evidence. She was also suggesting, based on a very biased survey of National Childbirth Trust enthusiasts, that episiotomies were infinitely worse in terms of maternal outcome than either spontaneous trauma, the perfect thing of course being an intact perineum, which I don't happen to believe, necessarily. But that did lend a lot of impetus and women did take notice and they started coming to the units in labour and would say, "Look, precisely what is going on? What are my choices?"' (interview with Jennifer Sleep).

Another example of the considerable influence wielded by Kitzinger in relation to the questioning of episiotomy has to do with the Department of Health discussions concerning inclusion of episiotomy in the Hospital Episode System (HES). HES is a data collection system which replaced the Maternity Hospital In-patient Enquiry (HIPE) which was abolished in 1985. According to a knowledgeable key informant, Department of Health officials insisted that there be no explicit question concerning episiotomy in HES as had been the case in HIPE. The reason for this was that they 'did not want to have reliable enough data to answer parliamentary questions on the subject arising out of Sheila Kitzinger's writings on the subject!' The omission of episiotomy from HES thus explains the lack of data on the national episiotomy rate since 1985. I confirmed that these data are indeed not available with an official in the Statistics Division of the Department of Health who responded to numerous inquiries for data on the use of episiotomy by stating, '... unfortunately the HES maternity data are of such poor quality that I am unable to supply you with any information' (R.A. Yeats, personal communication).

One final bit of evidence that Kitzinger's activities had not gone without notice comes from an unlikely source, H.M. Queen Elizabeth II. In 1982, Kitzinger was inducted by the Queen as a Member of the Order of the British Empire (MBE), the first person ever to be so honoured for anything to do with childbirth education. This accolade is an indication of not only Kitzinger's prominence in matters related to childbirth and the influence she exerts in this area but also societal acceptance of her work.

The continued questioning of episiotomy since 1985: a postscript

Since 1985 and the initial questioning of the practice of routine episiotomy, the operation has continued to be challenged by professionals and women and the evidence showing the procedure as not beneficial has continued accumulating.

In the decade between 1985 and 1995, over a dozen papers were published in the British midwifery literature questioning the practice. Most presented the mounting evidence disputing the presumed benefits of the operation and called on midwives to practise evidence-based midwifery (Maves, 1987; Sleep, 1987; Simpson, 1988; Moses, 1992). At least two systematic reviews of the literature were published in the midwifery periodical literature as well (Walker, 1990; Floud, 1994a).

A few papers presented the results of non-randomized prospective or retrospective studies. For example, Logue (1991) revealed that women experiencing episiotomy suffered greater perineal pain at twenty-four hours and five days postpartum and had no better pelvic floor muscular function than women experiencing a second-degree laceration or no perineal laceration at all. Another study found that women receiving an episiotomy had greater difficulty establishing sexual relations and greater postnatal perineal discomfort than women receiving no episiotomy (Kempster, 1986). Still other papers published during these years focused on some women's horrendous experiences with episiotomy (Kempster, 1987; Trevelyan, 1994) or on methods of avoiding an episiotomy (Cochrane, 1992; Floud, 1994b).

Another important source of ongoing midwifery questioning of episiotomy, which began in 1989, is the influential text *Myles Textbook for Midwives* (Bennett & Brown, 1989). The eleventh edition of the text was the first one after the retirement of Margaret Myles and, in the chapter entitled 'Physiology and management of the second stage of labour', exposes student midwives to the questioning of episiotomy and results of the West Bershire RCT (Sleep, 1989). The twelfth edition of the text published in 1993 continued to call on midwives to adopt a restrictive policy toward the use of episiotomy (Sleep, 1993).

Within medicine, questioning of episiotomy also persisted from the late 1980s through the 1990s. Differing somewhat from the earlier years when editorials and letters to the editor of journals predominated, the questioning that occurred after 1985 is more evidence-based. For example, during this period the results of two RCTs comparing the restrictive and liberal use of episiotomy and a three-year follow-up of the West Berkshire perineal management trial were reported. None of these studies found evidence to support the policy of liberal use of the operation or the claim that episiotomy healed better than a tear (House *et al.*, 1986, Argentine Episiotomy Trial Collaborative Group, 1993), prevented severe perineal trauma (Argentine Episiotomy Trial Collaborative Group, 1993), or prevented urinary incontinence from pelvic floor relaxation (Sleep & Grant, 1987).

Another four observational studies provided evidence that challenged the alleged prophylactic benefit that mediolateral episiotomy prevented severe perineal tears (Henriksen *et al.*, 1992; Anthony *et al.*, 1994; Sultan *et al.*, 1994; Fernando *et al.*, 1995). A fifth provided evidence that episiotomy was not without the potentially serious side effects of postpartum haemorrhage (Stones *et al.*, 1993). The rationales for performing episiotomy were also undermined in a review of the literature which offered recommendations for the management of low risk obstetric patients (Davis & Riedmann, 1990).

During these years there were also letters to the editors of the *British Journal of Obstetrics and Gynaecology*, the *BMJ*, and the *Lancet* which focused attention on episiotomy (Llewellyn-Jones, 1987; Griffiths, 1992; Friese *et al.*, 1993; Kuller *et al.*, 1994; Naugle *et al.*, 1994).

In the 1990s, the focus of the literature shifted from simply questioning the use of episiotomy and the benefits claimed of it to conducting research into the factors influencing the use of episiotomy and ways to reduce the prevalence of the operation. For example, at least two studies provided evidence that obstetricians are more likely to perform episiotomy than midwives. This observation persists when the medical conditions of the women being attended by these practitioners are taken into account. In other words, the difference between physicians and midwives is not because doctors see more high risk patients than midwives. Hundley *et al.* (1994) found that in their RCT comparing a midwifery unit with a traditional labour ward, obstetricians were more likely to perform the operation than midwives. Gerrits *et al.* (1994), in their retrospective cohort study, also found professional factors strongly related to the use of episiotomy; gynaecologists and registrars had episiotomy rates 3.4 and 2.5 times higher than midwives caring for comparable women.

Both these studies are important because they highlight that the use of episiotomy should be modifiable since they appear more related to professional training rather than obstetrical risk factors per se.

In a prospective observational study specifically designed to lower the use of episiotomy, Henriksen *et al.* (1994) recorded the use of episiotomy by 30 midwives for a period of 10 months and then provided each midwife with a graphical profile of her own and colleagues episiotomy rates. The use of episiotomy was then monitored for the next 19 months. The evaluation of the use of feedback by graphical profiles of rates of episiotomy revealed an absolute decline of 6.6% in the use of episiotomy during the second time period which persisted until the end of the study. In response to this paper, Stratton *et al.* (1995) at the Northwick Park Hospital, Harrow wrote to the editor of the *BMJ* about their mostly positive experience with using the same strategy of auditing midwifery practice and providing each midwife with awareness profiles. Their experience, however, suggested that continuous feedback was probably necessary to maintain the restrictive use of episiotomy.

Considering all the challenging of routine episiotomy that took place during the 1980s and early 1990s, by far the most authoritative and empirically based charge against the practice appeared in the new obstetrical textbook *Effective Care in Pregnancy and Childbirth (ECPC)* (Chalmers *et al.*, 1989). *ECPC* represented the most rigorous research synthesis ever undertaken in the area of obstetrics and maternity care. Each of the substantive chapters of the text present a systematic review and critical analysis of the relevant research and, where appropriate, a meta-analysis of existing RCTs. Originating from the National Perinatal Epidemiology Unit in Oxford, a majority of the 98 chapter authors are Canadian, American, Australian or European. The following quotation from a leading article in the *Medical Journal of Australia* places the importance of *ECPC* in context.

'From now on it will be impossible to write a leading article, to review the literature or to give an opinion on obstetric management without quoting from the Oxford Perinatal Data Base or its printed offspring *Effective Care in Pregnancy and Childbirth* by Chalmers *et al.* This arguably is the most important book ever to be written in the history of obstetrics' (MacLennan, 1990:1).

Specifically relating to the use of episiotomy, Sleep, Roberts and Chalmers, in their chapter on care during the second stage of labour, reported that there was 'no evidence ... that the liberal use of episiotomy reduces the risk of severe perineal trauma, improves perineal healing, prevents fetal trauma, or reduces the risk of urinary stress incontinence after delivery' (Sleep et al., 1989:1141). They advised that the practice of routine episiotomy should immediately be abandoned.

That same year, A Guide to Effective Care in Pregnancy and Childbirth (Enkin et al., 1989), a summarized paperback version of ECPC, was also released. The recommendation to abandon the routine use of episiotomy was repeated in this publication. In 1993, ECPC became an electronic journal called the Cochrane Collaboration: Pregnancy and Childbirth Database. The calls for the abandonment of episiotomy continued in the second edition of A Guide to Effective Care in Pregnancy and Childbirth (Enkin et al., 1995) published in 1995.

The impact of the ongoing questioning of episiotomy

As has already been described, national data on the use of episiotomy have not been collected since 1985 when episiotomy was deliberately removed from the HES by Department of Health officials. There is some evidence, however, from a national survey of 1493 mothers conducted in 1989 that 36% of women who gave birth vaginally that year received an episiotomy (Fleissig, 1993). This data suggests that the national episiotomy rate may not have declined between 1985 and 1989 despite the release of the results from the episiotomy RCTs in 1984 and episiotomy critiques which were published in the ensuing years.

There is also troubling data that the evidence-based pleas to abandon the routine use of episiotomy issued since 1989 in ECPC, A Guide to Effective Care in Pregnancy and Childbirth and the Cochrane Collaboration: Pregnancy and Childbirth Database probably did not prompt a continuing decline in the use of episiotomy by obstetricians. A 1993 survey of teaching and district hospitals in England revealed that only 79% of teaching hospitals and 51% of district hospitals had a copy of ECPC (Paterson-Brown et al., 1995). Even fewer institutions had the Oxford Database of Perinatal Trials, the forerunner of the Cochrane Collaboration: Pregnancy and Childbirth Database (62% of teaching hospitals and 16% of district hospitals). As long as evidence from meta-analysis of RCTs is not being widely used, there is little reason to think obstetrical practice will become more evidence-based.

Chapter 6

Challenging Routine Episiotomy in the USA

During approximately the same years that episiotomy was being challenged and used less frequently in the UK (1978–1985), the operation was also being challenged in the USA. However, the questioning of episiotomy there during these years did not result in a sudden appreciable decline in the operation's use as it did in the UK. In 1979, the first year that national statistics on episiotomy were collected in the USA, the operation was performed in 65.1% of all vaginal deliveries. As shown in Fig. 6, the use of episiotomy remained relatively stable for nearly a decade. By 1987, the national episiotomy rate had declined by only 4% to 61.1%. During the late 1980s through the 1990s episiotomy continued to be challenged and its use eventually

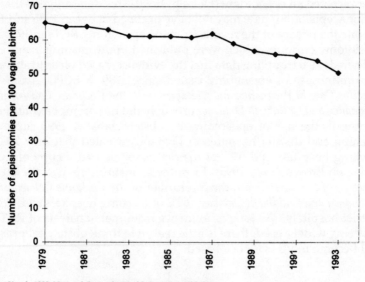

Source: Kozak, 1989; National Center for Health Statistics, 1992–95.

Fig. 6   National episiotomy rate for the USA (1979–1993).

started edging downward. Between 1987 and 1993, the episiotomy rate had declined to 50.4%, an absolute and relative decrease of 10.7% and 17.5% respectively.

Initial questioning of routine episiotomy by nurse-midwives

In the USA there are two types of midwives – nurse-midwives and lay midwives. Nurse-midwives receive formal training, are licensed to practise by the state and tend to practise in hospitals, birthing centres and in women's homes. In contrast, lay midwives are by and large unregulated and attend women almost exclusively in their homes. Nurse-midwives attend less than 5% of births in the USA.

It is important to remember that unlike midwives in the UK who have been legally recognized as independent practitioners since the enactment of the Midwives Act of 1902, nurse-midwifery in the USA is a relatively recent phenomenon. Midwifery in the USA was virtually abolished as a result of the successful lobbying efforts of American physicians at the turn of the century and it has only been since the 1970s that nurse-midwifery has been growing in popularity among childbearing women.

Regarding episiotomy, lay midwives report seldom performing the operation (Gaskin, 1977; Graham *et al.*, 1990). Being outside the 'official' maternity care system, they have had little need to question a practice they do not perform. Furthermore, they are much less organized than nurse-midwives in terms of using professional journals to transmit knowledge to their peers. For these reasons, this section focuses on the challenging of episiotomy by nurse-midwives.

The practice was first questioned by a nurse-midwife in the summer of 1977 in the *American Journal of Maternal and Child Nursing* (Anderson, 1977). In a major critique of childbirth practices, Anderson argued that the extension of obstetrical interventions designed for limited use with high risk labours to almost all labouring women was turning childbirth into a pathological event. She asserted that because birth was a physiologic process for most women, high levels of obstetric intervention were unnecessary and even damaging to mothers and infants. Referring to what she called the 'chain of events distorting childbirth' she suggested that interference in any part of the birth process had ramifications for later parts of the process.

Although criticizing the entire phenomenon of interventionist childbirth, episiotomy was one of the practices Anderson singled out. She hypothesized that the use of episiotomy was often precipitated by the earlier use of such routine procedures and practices as IVs, confining women to bed, induction, anaesthesia, forceps and lithotomy position (i.e. the 'cascade of intervention' effect). After presenting the commonly held beliefs about the prophylactic benefits of episiotomy, Anderson reported that there was little evidence to support any of these beliefs.

The following year at the annual convention of the National Student Nurses Association, controversy over episiotomy erupted. The student nurses debated the issue of episiotomy and passed a resolution 'opposing the unnecessary routine use of episiotomies for normal, spontaneous deliveries' (National Student Nurses Association, 1979:31). Within months, the controversy heightened with the publication of a review article on episiotomy. This paper appeared in the spring/summer issue of the *Journal of Nurse-Midwifery*, the official journal of the American College of Nurse-Midwives (Cogan & Edmunds, 1978), and was a republication of an article that appeared in an obstetrical journal the year before (Cogan & Edmunds, 1977). The paper reported that there was little scientific evidence for the prophylactic benefits claimed for episiotomy. The editorial board of the journal further ensured that the issue would receive a sound airing by soliciting comments on the paper from three nurse-midwives and a physician (Burkhardt, 1978; Elliott, 1978; Hartko, 1978; Phillips, 1978).

Many of the comments reveal that the commentators were reluctant to completely accept Cogan and Edmunds' reservations about routine episiotomy. Two of the writers were quite defensive. For example, the physician, while agreeing 'it is probably useful ... to re-examine various principles and techniques in any field' and 'that the justification for performing episiotomies requires further investigation', doubted if such an investigation would be possible (Hartko, 1978:22). The director of a nurse-midwifery service criticized Cogan and Edmunds for failing to indicate that under some circumstances episiotomy is necessary. She further attempted to discredit Cogan and Edmunds' findings by suggesting that their 'lack of medical knowledge and history' led them to use data 'too outdated to have a bearing on Modern Obstetrics' (Elliott, 1978:23). A second nurse-midwife stated that she did not support episiotomy as an established routine, yet ended up defending the practice based on her clinical experience and commonsense reasoning.

'One cannot resist thinking why repairs of pelvic floor muscles would be done if damage to these structures was not a reality, whether it was due to overstretching or tearing or even poor repair after episiotomy. Only the woman who has had this procedure done can truly say how revitalized she feels, and what a difference it has made to her sex life' (Phillips, 1978:22).

The only letter to completely support the questioning of episiotomy came from a nurse-midwife who was completing a PhD in Public Health. She emphasized the need for midwifery practice to be guided by sound research findings and called on midwives not only to 'raise questions but also to investigate them' (Burkhardt, 1978:23).

The questioning of episiotomy continued to mount as the first American evidence denying the claimed prophylactic benefits of epi- siotomy appeared. This evidence came from studies specifically designed to evaluate the alleged benefits of the operation. For example, at the third annual National Association of Parents and Professionals for Safe Alternatives in Childbirth (NAPSAC) conference in May 1978, Carol Brendsel, a registered nurse, and colleagues presented the results of a prospective study which matched 50 women who had received an episiotomy with 50 who had not. Contrary to established medical belief, analysis of the clinical examination data led these researchers to conclude that 'episiotomy is definitely not prophylactic against pelvic relaxation and is merely another factor in a large multifactorial process' (Brendsel *et al.*, 1979:174). This study, attained greater visibility when slightly modified versions of it were later published in *Women and Health*, a feminist journal devoted to women's health issues, and Sheila Kitzinger's *Episiotomy: Physical and Emotional Aspects* (Brendsel *et al.*, 1980; 1981).

Similar to that which occurred in the UK between 1979 and 1987, scepticism within the nurse-midwifery profession about the alleged benefits of episiotomy began gaining momentum. Nurse-midwifery critiques of episiotomy began mounting as did midwifery research refuting many of the age-old rationales for performing the operation. During this period, at least six nurse-midwifery master's research projects or theses were produced (e.g. Foss, 1977; Alden, 1979; Fischer, 1979; Schrag, 1979; Bowe, 1981; Triphen, 1983). In addition, 13 papers were published that questioned the routine use of episiotomy; 10 in the *Journal of Nurse-Midwifery*.

Among these papers were the results of one RCT, two non- randomized prospective studies, six retrospective studies of nurse- midwife attended births and three review articles. One study found that, contrary to the claim that episiotomy prevented third- and fourth- degree perineal lacerations, these lacerations were actually associated with the use of the operation (Fischer, 1979). Four studies investigated the claim that episiotomy prevented fetal injury. Again, contrary to obstetrical belief, none of the studies found that not preforming an episiotomy compromised the wellbeing of the baby (Bowe, 1981; Dunne, 1984; Roberts & Mokos Kriz, 1984; Formato, 1985). Two studies examined factors associated with perineal outcome or episiotomy (Cottrell & Shannahan, 1986; Nodine & Roberts, 1987). Another two showed that the prenatal practice of perineal massage decreased the need for episiotomy and the incidence of lacerations (Avery & Burket, 1986; Avery & Van Arsdale, 1987). Three additional critiques reviewed the literature for evidence of the presumed maternal benefits of episiotomy but found none (Schrag, 1979; Jennings, 1982; Bromberg, 1986). Finally, one other critique noted the controversy over the use of episiotomy and offered midwifery techniques for avoiding the need to perform the operation (Stiles, 1980).

Initial questioning of routine episiotomy by physicians

Just as in the UK, within medicine, questioning of the routine use of episiotomy was extremely infrequent in the USA prior to the 1980s. One of the earliest occasions at which routine episiotomy was publicly challenged was at the second conference of the NAPSAC in March 1977. NAPSAC is devoted to reforming and humanizing maternity services. At this conference, the rationale for performing routine episiotomy was disputed in papers presented by physicians Lewis Mehl and Herbert Ratner.

Mehl, a family physician, presented data on over 1000 homebirths which were matched with the same number of hospital births. In his analysis (Mehl, 1978b), Mehl empirically disputes claims made about the prophylactic benefits of the operation. The data revealed that episiotomy was performed significantly more often in hospital births than homebirths yet the incidence of third- and fourth-degree perineal lacerations was also significantly higher in births in hospital than at home. This finding was striking as prevention of these severe tears was one of the rationales for performing an episiotomy in the first place.

Ratner's paper, 'The history of the dehumanization of American medical practice', was more theoretical in nature and reviewed the origins of many routine American obstetrical interventions including episiotomy. This paper undermined routine obstetrical practices by suggesting that non-medical (i.e. non-scientific) factors greatly influenced obstetricians' adoption of episiotomy and other procedures in the early twentieth century. Ratner suggested that obstetricians advocated routine intervention for first-time mothers because:

- they had an ego-need to disassociate themselves from midwives;
- they made unwarranted extrapolations from the harm associated with some second stage labours to all primiparous deliveries;
- they did not take into account the risks associated with intervention;
- they accepted labour as a physiological process normative to all mammalia but singled out *Homo sapiens* as the species in which labour was pathologic;
- they refused to accept the multiparous state as normal;
- they disregarded the evidence of safety of homebirths for normal pregnancy in normal women; and
- they assumed but did not scientifically demonstrate the superiority

of routinized obstetric intervention over natural delivery (Ratner, 1978).

Because these papers were presented at essentially a homebirth conference, their dissemination was initially limited. Subsequently, however, the conference proceedings were published in book form with the title *21st Century Obstetrics Now!* (Stewart & Stewart, 1978). Neither this book, nor any of its chapters, was indexed in *Index Medicus* (the indexing system of the US National Library of Medicine) or MEDLINE (the computerized version of *Index Medicus*), making it inaccessible to the average physician. However, the material was known to the small minority of professionals involved in the childbirth reform movement of the 1970s. In total, after two printings, 7000 copies of the book were printed.

An earlier version of Mehl's paper entitled 'Home birth versus hospital birth: comparisons of outcomes of matched populations' was also presented at the 104th Annual Meeting of the American Public Health Association in October 1976. His homebirth research gained wider exposure when it was presented in articles published in *Women and Health* (1977–78) and the *Journal of Reproductive Medicine* (1977), and as a chapter in Kitzinger and Davis' *The Place of Birth* (1978a).

In April 1977, the first paper to question the practice of routine episiotomy in the obstetrical literature appeared in *Contemporary OB/GYN*. This paper, provocatively titled 'The unkindest cut of all?' reviewed the literature for evidence supporting the alleged advantages of the operation and also examined the evidence relating to known episiotomy side effects. The authors, both psychologists, concluded that:

'...although episiotomy may somewhat reduce the laceration rate and shorten the second stage of labor, it may also have unsatisfactory anatomic results and lead to increased blood loss and postpartum and coital pain. We found little evidence that episiotomy improves or maintains the condition of the pelvic floor and no evidence that it reduces the likelihood of cystocele or rectocyle or improves sexual functioning after birth ... Perhaps what is most striking about the literature on episiotomy is the absence of clear evidence as to the advantage of the procedure. We have found no data showing a positive relationship between episiotomy and subsequent maternal or infant health in births that are not forceps-assisted ... Review of the episiotomy literature might lead to increasingly conservative and thoughtful use of the procedure' (Cogan & Edmunds, 1977:60).

Despite challenging a procedure that had been well entrenched for decades, this paper prompted only three letters to the editor. Not surprisingly, two of them expressed dismay that the routine use of episiotomy was even being questioned (Eichner, 1977; Hyams, 1977).

The third supported the conclusions reached by Cogan and Edmunds and praised the journal for publishing this 'heretical' article (Newton, 1977).

This episiotomy critique had little impact on the broader obstetrical community. *Contemporary OB/GYN* is a relatively unknown and marginal 'throw-away' obstetrical journal distributed without charge. It has a low circulation, less than 13 000 in 1990, and was not indexed in *Index Medicus* or MEDLINE. This not only indicates the lower status of this journal but reflects the limited dissemination of papers published in it. In an age when computerized searches of the medical literature are so heavily relied upon to locate literature on topics of interest, papers published in journals not indexed on MEDLINE tend to be overlooked. Ironically, Cogan and Edmunds' paper would have been completely ignored by physicians had it not been for the response it received from the sixteenth edition of *Williams Obstetrics*. Intending to discredit and silence those daring enough to question routine episiotomy, the editors of this textbook, by citing Cogan and Edmunds, actually helped publicize their paper among obstetricians, or at the very least, among medical students (even if in a negative way).

'More recently, the advantages provided by episiotomy have been questioned by some individuals (Cogan & Edmunds, 1977), as have most aspects of obstetric care. It can be said with certainty that, since the era of in-hospital deliveries with episiotomy, there has been an appreciable decrease in the number of women subsequently hospitalized for treatment of symptomatic cystocele, rectocele, uterine prolapse, and stress incontinence!' (Pritchard & MacDonald, 1980:430).

Between 1977 and 1980, medical questioning of routine episiotomy was practically non-existent. The issue was not raised again until 1981 when family practitioners in both the USA and Canada simultaneously called for a critical appraisal of the management of normal labour and delivery. In the *Journal of Family Practice*, Brody and Thompson (1981) published an important critique of what they called the 'maximin [sic] strategy in modern obstetrics'. They described this strategy as 'making the best of the worst possible outcome, regardless of the actual probability of that outcome occurring' (i.e. treating all patients as though something might go wrong and taking action to prevent this possible negative outcome before it occurred) (Brody & Thompson, 1981:977). Brody and Thompson contend that many accepted obstetrical practices and interventions, including prophylactic episiotomy, exemplify this maximin strategy despite there being little research documenting superior clinical results when this strategy is used. In questioning the routine use of episiotomy, Brody and Thompson reported:

'Studies demonstrate the safety of midline episiotomy and episio-proctotomy, but have not documented the need for episiotomy of any sort in the first place. This lack of documentation is striking given the wide disparity between the 80 percent episiotomy rate in standard obstetrical units and the nearly zero percent rate among some midwives, who emphasize a slower second stage of labor, careful control of the descending part, and perineal massage. However, the question whether acceptance of a slow second stage places the fetus at greater risk leads directly to the question of instrumental delivery, and early episiotomy is a necessary concomitant of most instrumental approaches' (Brody & Thompson, 1981:982).

In a similar type of discussion piece in the *Canadian Medical Association Journal*, Schneider (1981), a family practitioner, also called for a re-evaluation of maternity care. Supporting the 'humanization of the birth process', he too reviewed the evidence for routine or common hospital practices. Schneider disputed the 'usual belief' that episiotomy decreased the risk of pelvic relaxation and perineal tears by citing studies by Mehl (1977) and Chalmers *et al.* (1976b).

The first critique of episiotomy in the obstetrical literature written by an obstetrician appeared in 1982 in the highly respected journal *Obstetrical and Gynecological Survey*. In a note appended to a condensation of a British article on postepisiotomy pain, Edward Stewart Taylor, editor-in-chief of the journal and a past president of the AAOG (1971) and past vice-president of the AGS (1975), wrote:

'When labor is normal and delivery spontaneous, episiotomy is usually not required. There will soon be a review article appearing in the *Survey* which discusses the use and overuse of episiotomy. The procedure has not been scientifically tested to determine its true indications. The procedure has been classified as routine for primiparous deliveries, but it is debatable that it has all the virtues attributed to it, such as preservation of the perineum and prevention of rectocele and cystocele ... I think that patients who have a normal spontaneous vertex delivery usually do not benefit from episiotomy' (Taylor, 1982).

It was not until the following year, however, that the questioning of episiotomy was brought undeniably into obstetrical circles with the publication of the review article Taylor anticipated. This important paper presented the results of an American government sponsored study of the risks and benefits of episiotomy (Thacker & Banta, 1983). Authored by Stephen Thacker, a physician and Director of the Division of Surveillance and Epidemiologic Studies at the Centers for Disease Control in Atlanta, and David Banta, also a physician and Assistant Director of Health and the Life Sciences Division of the US Office of Technology Assessment in Washington, this publication was the first truly exhaustive review of the English language episiotomy literature from 1860 to 1980. Upon reviewing over 350 books and articles,

Thacker and Banta uncovered considerable evidence of risks associated with the episiotomy (pain, dyspareunia, oedema and infection), but found 'no clearly defined evidence for its efficacy, particularly for routine use' (1983:322). Regarding the then widely accepted medical allegations that episiotomy prevented perineal, pelvic relaxation or fetal brain damage, Thacker and Banta reported:

'Overall, these studies do not indicate that episiotomy offers a clear benefit to women in terms of decreased numbers of lacerations ... Clearly, none of the studies have adequately analyzed the relationship of episiotomy to lacerations' (Thacker & Banta, 1983:327).

'Although the prevention of long-term damage to the pelvic floor and interference with sexual function are frequently cited as reasons for episiotomy, there are few data to support or refute this clinical hypothesis' (Thacker & Banta, 1983:327) ... 'In summary, the role of episiotomy in preventing serious pelvic relaxation has not been adequately studied' (Thacker & Banta, 1983:328).

'As with other possible benefits of episiotomy, little data exist to support the utilization of the procedure to prevent cerebral damage to the fetus, and no follow-up studies of infants have been designed to address this particular issue' (Thacker & Banta, 1983:329).

Based on these findings, Thacker and Banta recommended that physicians restrict their use of episiotomy. In much the same way as Kitzinger had done in the UK two years earlier, Thacker and Banta challenged the obstetric community to practise evidence-based medicine and prove episiotomy beneficial in adequately designed clinical trials.

Despite undertaking the most comprehensive review of the evidence relating to the risks and benefits of episiotomy to date, this paper failed to generate much controversy or debate about episiotomy within American obstetrics. As had occurred with Cogan and Edmunds' (1977) questioning of episiotomy, the seventeenth edition of *Williams Obstetrics* (Pritchard *et al.*, 1985) acknowledged Thacker and Banta's analysis and then dismissed it. The only difference between the sixteenth and seventeenth editions of the text was that the reference to Cogan and Edmunds was replaced by one to Thacker and Banta. According to Banta, very little interest was shown in their work on episiotomy which contrasted sharply with that which had occurred after an earlier review they had done on the benefits and risks of electronic fetal monitoring.

'One of my greatest disappointments professionally has been the limited impact of this paper. In contrast to the EFM paper, it got little attention. One or the other of us did present it in a number of places. There was little criticism this time, little controversy... Physicians showed little interest in our work. Although we had much loud criticism of our EFM work, we had some rather impressive congratulations, and a number of quiet encouragements from physicians concerned about the issue. In the episiotomy case, I don't remember any physician interest at all, except for Murray Enkin... So I just felt that across the board, it just fell flat, completely flat' (interview with David Banta).

Outside of medicine, however, the paper was widely disseminated within the childbirth and women's health movement. The paper in *Obstetrical and Gynecological Survey* was in fact the third to be published by Thacker and Banta. They first presented the results of the review at the 'Technological Approaches to Obstetrics: Benefits, Risks, Alternatives' conference in October 1981. The following spring, this presentation was published in the journal *Birth. Issues in Perinatal Care and Education* (Banta & Thacker, 1982). Also in 1982, another slightly modified version of the paper appeared in the journal *Women and Health* (Thacker & Banta, 1982). Furthermore, the article published in *Women and Health* was included in Young's 1983 book *Obstetrical Intervention and Technology in the 1980s* and the article in *Birth* was reprinted in Kitzinger and Simkin's *Episiotomy and the Second Stage of Labor* (1984; 1986).

In total, the original three papers by Thacker and Banta prompted only one letter to the editor of *Birth*. Similar to some of the responses to Cogan and Edmund's (1977; 1978) paper, the letter vehemently defended routine episiotomy (Papst, 1982:268). In essence, the letter from a physician simply stated that he believed the claims made about the operation were true and that it mattered little to him that there was no evidence supporting them.

In September 1983, the second ever episiotomy critique written by an American obstetrician appeared in *Obstetrics and Gynecology* (Goodlin, 1983). In the section of the journal that is devoted to commentaries called 'After office hours', Goodlin of the Department of Obstetrics and Gynecology at the University of Nebraska Medical Center briefly reviewed the literature on methods of protecting the perineum during childbirth and described his own birthing room experience. His conclusion was that prophylactic episiotomy was not indicated.

What appears to be the first empirical US study published in the American obstetrical literature to raise questions about the rationale for performing episiotomy appeared in *Obstetrics and Gynecology* in 1984. The retrospective matching study comparing midwifery care with physician care of women in labour revealed that the health of mothers and infants was not compromised when midwives did not routinely perform episiotomy (Baruffi et al., 1984). The following year, a review of the literature on sexuality in pregnancy and the puerperium published in *Obstetrical and Gynecological Survey* highlighted the suspected relationship between the use of episiotomy and postpartum dyspareunia (painful sexual intercourse) (Reamy & White, 1985).

In 1986, Edward Stewart Taylor, editor of *Obstetrical and Gynecological Survey*, drew attention to an observational study originally published in the *British Journal of Obstetrics and Gynaecology* (Buekens *et al.*, 1985) which showed that mediolateral episiotomy did not appear to prevent severe perineal lacerations as claimed. Taylor used this opportunity to cite Thacker and Banta's (1983) review article and declared that 'there is no proof that any of the [alleged] benefits occur from episiotomy when the patient has a normal spontaneous vaginal delivery of a full-term infant in occipitoanterior position' (Taylor, 1986:231).

The same year, in the *Journal of Reproductive Medicine*, obstetricians from the University of Cincinnati Medical Clinic reported the results of a retrospective study of over 2600 vaginal deliveries which indicated that, contrary to obstetrical belief, episiotomy was not prophylactic for severe perineal lacerations (Gass *et al.*, 1986). They reported that 'the results of the study do not support routine use of episiotomy' and recommended the more selective use of episiotomy. Also during the summer of 1986, Michael Varner, an obstetrician from the University of Iowa Hospitals, published a review article in *Clinical Obstetrics and Gynecology* in which he presented the evidence for the claims made for episiotomy and concluded that, 'episiotomy should not be performed routinely' (Varner, 1986:315).

In 1987, Edward Stewart Taylor again questioned the practice of routine episiotomy in an editorial note appended to an article about repair of episiotomy abstracted in *Obstetrical and Gynecological Survey*. In his note, Taylor (1987) reported that episiotomy was often performed unnecessarily and again cited Thacker and Banta's review.

Also in 1987, Thorp *et al.* (1987) reported in *Obstetrics and Gynecology* on an interesting prospective non-randomized controlled study of 379 women. This study set out to determine the effect of restricting the use of episiotomy to operative vaginal deliveries and/or cases of fetal distress. The study design called for one resident physician (registrar) to perform only 'selective' episiotomy on his patients while his fellow residents performed episiotomy at their own discretion to limit perineal trauma. The study found that severe lacerations were significantly less frequent when the use of episiotomy was restricted and that no one had a severe laceration without an episiotomy. Thorp and colleagues interpreted the results of the study to 'suggest that episiotomy is a factor in the occurrence of third- and fourth-degree perineal lacerations' and concluded 'it would seem prudent to re-evaluate its [episiotomy's] routine use' (Thorp *et al.*, 1987:262).

Creating a climate conducive to professional questioning

When the early professional questioning of routine episiotomy is placed within a societal context, it is clear that pressure responsible for precipitating the production of these critiques came largely from outside nurse-midwifery or medicine. Similar to that which occurred in the UK, this pressure came from prominent childbirth reformers and childbearing women. It also came from another source which had not been present in the UK, the women's health movement. Though the sources of pressure were different in the US, the effect was the same. Just as in the UK, these individuals and organizations raised lay and professional consciousness of episiotomy by helping to transform it into a collective or social issue. This consciousness raising involved airing doubts about the obstetric rationale for performing the operation and drawing attention to its adverse effects. The effect of lay questioning of episiotomy was to generate uncertainty. This produced a climate in which sympathetic health professionals felt justified, in some cases even compelled, to investigate the lay claims and produce their own critiques of the practice for professional consumption.

The earliest comprehensive lay questioning of episiotomy was published five years before professionals began writing their episiotomy critiques. In 1972 Doris Haire, nationally recognized 'as the foremost American lobbyist for pregnant women and their unborn children' (Edwards & Waldorf, 1984:109), published a special report on American childbirth practices for the International Childbirth Education Association (ICEA) (Haire, 1972). The 30-page monograph containing 102 references to the scientific literature was called *The Cultural Warping of Childbirth*. Haire, co-president of the ICEA in 1972, wrote this monograph because she was troubled by America's relatively high infant mortality rates compared with other industrialized countries, and what she considered the staggering incidence of neurological impairment among American children and adults.

To find explanations for these phenomena, Haire visited 30 countries observing their obstetric techniques and procedures and interviewing physicians, midwives and parents. Evaluating all the obstetrical practices performed during a typical American delivery, Haire concluded that the high rates of infant mortality and neurological impairment were attributable to interventionist obstetrics which had a '...tendency to warp the birth experience, distorting it into a pathological event, rather than a physiological one, for the normal childbearing woman' (Haire, 1972:7). In all, Haire considered the scientific evidence for nearly two-dozen routine American obstetrical procedures, one of which being episiotomy. Calling into doubt the usual medical rationales for episiotomy, she reported:

'There is no research or evidence to indicate that routine episiotomy reduces the incidence of pelvic relaxation (structural damage to the pelvic floor musculature) in the mother. Nor is there any research or evidence that routine episiotomy reduces neurological impairment in the child who has shown no signs of fetal distress or that the procedure helps maintain subsequent male or female sexual response' (Haire, 1972:20).

At the time and for years afterwards, *The Cultural Warping of Childbirth* was responsible for drawing attention to American childbirth practices, including episiotomy. Haire's monograph was widely distributed. It was initially released in 1972 and reprinted in a special issue of *Environmental Child Health* in June 1973. It also served as a book chapter in *The Cultural Crisis of Modern Medicine* edited by Ehrenreich (Haire, 1978) and was reprinted by the ICEA in 1976 with a postscript. Because it was still in demand, it was reprinted again nine years later. Furthermore, most experts in the fields of maternity care and childbirth education agree that the monograph had a tremendous impact on maternity care and providers of maternity care.

'...[the] monograph was so influential that it altered forever the way in which American birth customs were regarded by critics and reformers. Many observers had criticized one procedure or another in labor and birth protocols, but no one had placed all components of an average hospital birth in chronological order together with their justification and outcome. Few had articulated how much such a pattern of intervention distorted the physiology of childbirth so that it was transferred into pathology. And none had had the inspiration to name the pattern by its accumulated effect: The Cultural Warping of Childbirth' (Edwards & Waldorf, 1984:109).

The routine use of episiotomy received more exposure in 1973, when the women's health movement came out strongly against the practice. In *Our Bodies, Ourselves. A Book by and for Women*, the first handbook of the women's health movement, the Boston Women's Health Book Collective (1973) rejected routine episiotomy.

'Although episiotomies are done routinely in the United States, there is often no need for them. If the mother is unanesthetized, she will feel when to stop pushing and when to start easing her baby gently out. Her doctor can direct her. The vaginal opening can stretch to very wide proportions without tearing.'

'We question the practice of administering episiotomies to all women before delivery' (Boston Women's Health Book Collective, 1973:187).

While the Boston Women's Health Book Collective (1973:187) was willing to agree that it made sense for a doctor to perform an episiotomy to either 'avoid a possible ragged-edged tear in the perineum or to ensure the birth of the baby as speedily as possible', they were less convinced of the arguments that episiotomy prevented pelvic relaxation or improved sexual functioning. Indeed, they found the idea of episiotomies being performed for men's sexual pleasure extremely offensive.

> 'Often male doctors are concerned that the woman's looser vagina will interfere with the man's sexual pleasure during intercourse.
>
> [quoting a woman] 'I saw my doctor at the checkup six weeks after my baby was born. Full of male pride, he told me during my pelvic exam, "I did a beautiful job sewing you up. You're as tight as a virgin; your husband should thank me" (Boston Women's Health Book Collective, 1973:187).

There is little doubt that the questioning of routine episiotomy by the Boston Women's Health Book Collective greatly popularized women's discontent with the indiscriminate use of the operation. By 1976, when a second revised edition of *Our Bodies, Ourselves* was issued, over one-million copies of the first edition had already been sold (Ruzek, 1978:32). Furthermore, the anti-episiotomy sentiments expressed in the 1973 edition were repeated in the 1976 edition.

The questioning of the routine use of episiotomy was brought once more before the American public in the spring of 1975, with the publication of Arms' bestseller *Immaculate Deception* (Arms, 1975a). This book took issue with the medicalization of childbirth, and episiotomy was one of many obstetrical practices Arms discussed. In much the same way as Haire had done several years earlier, Arms presented the medical rationales that physicians had tended to put forward for performing episiotomy and then skilfully discredited each one using commonsense arguments, anecdotal evidence, statistics and whatever other evidence she could find.

This book had wide exposure; it was first published by Houghton Mifflin in May 1975, with a second printing in June. It was subsequently published by Bantam in June 1977, with a second printing in December 1979 and a third in October 1981 (Arms, 1981). In addition, the book was serialized in the *San Francisco Chronicle-Examiner* in April, and in the journal *Prevention* in May 1975. Arms' questioning of routine episiotomy also figured prominently in an article she wrote for *Ms* magazine in May 1975 (Arms, 1975b).

The lay questioning and undermining of the medical rationales for performing episiotomy increased and became fairly extensive during the early and mid 1970s. In addition to the criticism from Haire, Arms and the Boston Women's Health Book Collective, challenges to routine episiotomy also appeared in popular childbirth education books directed at expectant parents. For example, in her book *Methods of Childbirth: A Complete Guide to Childbirth Classes and Maternity Care*,

Constance Bean (1972), a co-founder of the Boston Association for Childbirth Education and a pioneer in family-centred maternity, critically discussed the routine use of episiotomy in hospitals and challenged the practice. Similarly, Lester Hazell (1976), a past co-president of the ICEA, questioned the routine use of episiotomy and disputed the medical rationales for performing the operation in her popular book *Commonsense Childbirth*.

Furthermore, doubts about the need for routine episiotomy had become so common in lay circles that by the mid 1970s the questioning of routine episiotomy could be found in mainstream or traditional women's magazines. For example, some childbirth articles that disputed the alleged prophylactic benefits of episiotomy appeared in such popular magazines as *Good Housekeeping* (Yunker, 1975:58), *McCall's* (Lake, 1976; Pascoe, 1977) and *Women's Day* (Davis, 1976).

Throughout the 1980s, the lay questioning of episiotomy persisted. Articles appeared in women's and childbirth magazines which were totally devoted to episiotomy or included a section that discussed the operation. Some of these articles challenged the practice of routine episiotomy or, at the very least, described the controversy surrounding it (e.g. Yarrow, 1982; Hillard, 1984; Shea, 1985; Toal, 1986; Lieberman, 1989; Longo, 1989); others presented ways to avoid the operation (e.g. MacCallum, 1982); and still others drew attention to the side effects of the operation (e.g. Gaylin, 1982).

As the number of best-selling childbirth education books began increasing during the 1980s, so did the questioning of episiotomy. In these books, usually in the chapter describing hospital procedures, the medical rationales for episiotomy were presented along with the lack of evidence for each (e.g. Bean, 1982; Inch, 1982; Young, 1982; Young, 1983; Brackbill *et al.*, 1984; Elkins, 1985). The Boston Women's Health Book Collective (1984) continued to question the practice in *The New Our Bodies, Ourselves*. Harrison (1982), in her book *A Woman in Residence*, described her experiences going through an obstetrics and gynaecology residency training programme, raised questions about the practice and described physicians' resistance to limiting its use.

Another significant source of challenging in the USA was Sheila Kitzinger. In 1984, Kitzinger with Penny Simkin, an American physical therapist and childbirth educator, edited a book entitled *Episiotomy and the Second Stage of Labor* (Kitzinger & Simkin, 1984). The book began as the American edition of *Episiotomy. Physical and Emotional Aspects*, which Kitzinger (1981) edited for the NCT in the UK. At 135 pages long, it contains both a collection of critiques on episiotomy and the second stage of labour and advice on how to conduct the second stage so as to minimize the need for the operation. *Episiotomy and the Second Stage of Labor* was at the time and still is the only English language book devoted exclusively to influencing second stage management practices and reducing the use of episiotomy.

As a result of the interest shown in the book, a new edition appeared in 1986 (Kitzinger & Simkin, 1986). It remained the same except for the addition of a chapter that reviewed the research findings on episiotomy and management of the second stage which had been published since the release of the first edition two years earlier, most importantly the results of the RCTs of episiotomy.

Kitzinger was also involved in the lay questioning of episiotomy in the USA and Canada in other ways as well. From very early on, she and Swenson of *Our Bodies, Ourselves* had a close relationship and exchanged information on all aspects of childbirth including episiotomy. Kitzinger also influenced the American questioning of episiotomy through her position as consultant to the ICEA (an organization based in the USA). In fact, in her capacity as consultant, Kitzinger authored an *ICEA Review* (a newsletter) devoted to the issue of episiotomy in August 1985. Following a commentary in which she noted the lack of research on episiotomy and its sequelae and questioned the evidence for the routine use of episiotomy, Kitzinger presented abstracts of a number of research articles on the topic as well as her own writings on episiotomy. Later on, Kitzinger also brought the questioning of routine episiotomy directly to the attention of women through the very popular American editions of her books on pregnancy and childbirth (Kitzinger, 1987; 1988).

During the 1970s and early 1980s, there was yet another source of non-health professional questioning of episiotomy. The controversy over the routine use of episiotomy was also raised in more academic works dealing with the history of childbirth and childbirth practices. During discussions of typical American obstetrical practices, a few pages are usually devoted to describing DeLee's influence on the development of routine episiotomy in the USA and Canada and the lack of evidence justifying the practice. The unproven benefits of episiotomy are noted in such works as Wertz and Wertz's *Lying-in: A History of Childbirth in America* (1979:141–3, 183–4; 1989:141–3, 183–4), Romalis' *Childbirth: Alternatives to Medical Control* (1981:76, 150–151), Edwards and Waldorf's *Reclaiming Birth: History and Heroines of American Childbirth Reform* (1984:142–5), Katz Rothman's *Giving Birth: Alternatives in Childbirth* (1984:58–61), Arney's *Power and the Profession of Obstetrics* (1985:69–75) and Leavitt's *Brought to Bed: Childbearing in America 1750–1950* (1986:179–180).

As for childbearing women, there is some evidence they too were questioning the need for routine episiotomy. For example, Hazell's mid-1970s study of homebirths reveals that the desire to avoid episiotomies was one of the main reasons given by couples for choosing a homebirth over a hospital birth (Hazell, 1974; 1975). A similar finding was also reported in an article in *Women's Day* (Maynard, 1977). A number of other papers and articles also suggest that consumer interest during the 1970s and 1980s in midwifery care and alternative birth centres was prompted in part by women who wanted to avoid routine episiotomies (e.g. Norwood, 1978; Randal, 1979; Goodlin, 1983). A 1979 survey of Washington State hospitals revealed that the presence of alternative birth rooms was associated with more delivery options. One of these options was no episiotomy (Dobbs & Shy, 1981). Furthermore, it is not uncommon to find reports, such as the following, that allude to women's desire to avoid episiotomies.

'Women who have attended childbirth classes realize that an episiotomy is necessary in some deliveries, but ask, "Why must it always be done?"' (Lake, 1976:129).

'While North America probably leads the world in its acceptance of routine episiotomy, in the last decade we have seen and heard women protesting what they interpret as a thoughtless disregard for this highly sensuous and sexual part of their bodies' (Simkin, 1986:4).

'Women are requesting intact perineums with delivery' (Nodine & Roberts, 1987:123).

There is also evidence from at least two prominent American obstetricians representing the obstetrical establishment that women during the 1970s and 1980s were demanding the avoidance of having episiotomies. For example, Danforth, during his presidential address before the AGS in 1974, presented the many accomplishments of DeLee including the prophylactic forceps and episiotomy operation. He repeated DeLee's now famous claims that prophylactic episiotomy and forceps prevented damage to women's pelvic soft parts and spared babies' brains from injury. He then said parenthetically:

'...it is disconcerting to some of us, and at times even grotesque, to observe the increasing numbers of modern women who demand spontaneous delivery, and whose obstetricians comply, regardless of the length of time the fetal head must pound against the pelvic floor' (Danforth, 1974:581).

Similar comments were echoed a decade later by Robert Wilson, a past president of the AGS, in an editorial in *Postgraduate Medicine* on the effects of consumerism in obstetric care. Wilson commented:

'A further example of an area where physicians may have given away too much in responding to patient pressure is use of the episiotomy, which is popularly considered unnecessary, even for primigravidas' (Wilson, 1984:25).

That Danforth and Wilson felt the need to defend episiotomy and publicly censure their colleagues for bowing to patient demand suggests that the questioning of episiotomy was having an effect at some level.

Furthermore, on one rare occasion, consumer preferences concerning routine episiotomy were actually quantified in a scientific manner. A 1977 survey of a random sample of 694 Boulder City mothers found that 78% did not want an episiotomy unless absolutely necessary (Pascoe, 1977). If the results of this survey are generalisable to the population, women's opposition to routine episiotomy in the late 1970s may have been considerable.

The influence of childbirth reformers on professional questioning

It is strongly evident that the professionals who were writing the early episiotomy critiques were often responding to, or, at the very least, receptive to, the lay challenge of routine episiotomy. Lay questioning of episiotomy was an antecedent to the professional questioning of the practice. This is demonstrated in the fact that the writings of prominent lay childbirth reformers such as Haire and Arms were cited by some of the earliest professional critics. Typically, Haire and Arms' writings were referenced as evidence that the alleged prophylactic benefits of episiotomy were not supported by research (e.g. Anderson, 1977; Mehl, 1977; Mehl, 1977–78; Schrag, 1979; Brendsel *et al.*, 1980; Bowe, 1981; Brody & Thompson, 1981; Banta & Thacker, 1982; Jennings, 1982; Thacker & Banta, 1982; 1983; Bromberg, 1986). As professionals are often reluctant to admit being influenced by outsiders, their willingness to cite lay sources suggests they must have found the lay questioning somewhat compelling. This can be seen in many of the professional critiques dating from the late 1970s through the 1980s, as the following passages reveal:

'Although we find wide medical acceptance of episiotomy, there are arguments against the procedure in contemporary literature, particularly from the growing women's health consciousness movement. In popular books, such as *Our Bodies, Ourselves*, women have questioned the practice of routinely performing episiotomies during the second stage... We should expect to find some compelling arguments in favor of a procedure that has been so widely accepted in this country but about which a muted disagreement seems to be emerging...' (Cogan & Edmunds, 1977:56).

'Growing consumer interest is forcing the questioning of routine episiotomy' (Stiles, 1980:106).

'Routine episiotomy is being called into question by patients. Several articles have appeared in women's magazines about unnecessary episiotomies, and the subject has been discussed on radio and television talk shows' (Taylor, 1982).

In a few cases, the professional critiques actually state that lay challenging of episiotomy was responsible for their designing and implementing studies to scientifically evaluate the benefits claimed of episiotomy (e.g. Fischer, 1979; Avery & Burket, 1986).

Clearly the continuous and increasing challenging of episiotomy by prominent childbirth reformers and childbearing women during the 1970s and early 1980s created a climate in which a small number of professionals (more nurse-midwives than physicians) were prompted to question the practice themselves. There are also examples where this challenging influenced the professional questioning of episiotomy more directly. Haire, for example, was instrumental in bringing about the first prospective matching study which evaluated the allegation that episiotomy was prophylactic against subsequent pelvic relaxation. This study, which was carried out by Brendsel *et al.* (1979; 1980; 1981), matched 50 women who had received an episiotomy with 50 women who had not. The study found no significant differences between the two groups in the incidence of postpartum gynaecological problems, thus providing data discrediting the well-established medical belief that episiotomy was prophylactic for pelvic relaxation.

Haire not only encouraged the decision to conduct the research (Brendsel *et al.*, 1979:169), she also supported the project financially. The study was partially funded by a grant from the American Foundation For Maternal and Child Health. Haire is president and founder of this foundation, which she set up to fund '"counterstream" research, outside the popular interventionist trends in childbirth' (Edwards & Waldorf, 1984:115).

Another example of research being motivated by childbirth reformers is Banta and Thacker's literature review of the risks and benefits of episiotomy (1982). The decision to evaluate episiotomy was greatly influenced by Norma Swenson, one of the editors of *Our Bodies, Ourselves*. Banta was looking for another procedure to study and Swenson during several discussions proposed episiotomy. Banta also acknowledges receiving considerable help from Kitzinger and Haire. Haire and her Foundation, for example, were directly responsible for the timely publication of their paper in *Obstetrical and Gynecological Survey* (Thacker & Banta, 1983). By paying a subsidy, she ensured the paper was published a year earlier than it would otherwise have been.

Professional concerns: staking out turf

Another stimulus that fuelled early professional questioning of episiotomy was related to the inter-professional concerns of nurse-midwives and the intra-professional concerns of family physicians. For both these groups, interest in the questioning of episiotomy was related to attempts to resist obstetrical control and provide justification for deviating from the obstetrical norm of routine episiotomy.

Nurse-midwifery is a profession dedicated to patient satisfaction and reduction of the use of unnecessary interventions (Avery & Burket, 1986:134). During the 1970s and 1980s, it was also a relatively new health care profession seeking widespread recognition from both the public and obstetric communities. For nurse-midwives, not performing routine episiotomy, a hallmark of their profession, differentiated the maternity care they provided from that provided by obstetricians. For some childbearing women, this was a primary reason for wanting to be attended by a nurse-midwife as opposed to an obstetrician. The avoidance of episiotomy, however, posed a dilemma for a nurse-midwifery profession struggling to gain legitimacy. Not performing routine episiotomy involved going against obstetric orthodoxy, thereby exposing the profession to medical criticism at a very vulnerable period in its development.

Many of the nurse-midwifery critiques of episiotomy were written with the intent of remedying this dilemma. By using original nurse-midwifery research to challenge the obstetrical rationales behind routine episiotomy, the critiques were to show that the nurse-midwifery practice of avoiding routine episiotomy was evidence-based and defensible. In effect, it was part of an effort to develop a scientific body of nurse-midwifery knowledge which could be used to justify non-interventionist nurse-midwifery practices to both physicians and the public. The following passages show that some nurse-midwives were keenly aware of their profession's vulnerability to consumer demand and its tenuous professional status in relation to medicine.

'For long periods midwives had not been allowed to perform or repair episiotomies. For this and other reasons many midwives became skilled at delivering babies over intact perineums with minor or no lacerations. Today many maternity patients are beginning to ask midwives not to use episiotomies. Midwives are torn between accepted standards of medical practice and the wishes of their clients and traditional approaches of midwifery practice. Nurse-midwives must begin to seek information about the causes of perineal tears and the best methods of protecting the pelvic floor tissues' (Fischer, 1979:19).

'One of the newest requests is to deliver without an episiotomy. This request is controversial and is awkward for birth attendants. Should they comply with accepted medical standards or with the wishes of their clients? Nurse-midwives are especially affected by this controversy. Because the profession is still gaining acceptance in the American medical community, the actions of nurse-midwives are often highly scrutinized' (Dunne, 1984:29).

Although the role of general practitioners in American maternity care was considerably more established than that of nurse-midwives, the development of the specialty of family practice, with family practice residency training, did not occur until the 1970s. In family practice, emphasis is placed on the family as a psychological unit and the assessment of individual emotional needs, making client satisfaction an important outcome (Brody & Thompson, 1981). By capitalizing on the public's dissatisfaction with traditional obstetrical care, the questioning of routine episiotomy by family practitioners in the early 1980s provided the newly developing specialty with an opportunity to advance its own agenda. As some family physicians observed:

'Maternal satisfaction with the labor and delivery experience is an important goal in itself in addition to whatever it may contribute to the bonding process. Maternal dissatisfaction plays a major role in the current public criticism of obstetrical practices, and in the push for more maternity center care...' (Brody & Thompson, 1981:983).

Furthermore, like nurse-midwives, the questioning of episiotomy by family physicians during the early 1980s was also part of an effort to stake claim to low risk, non-interventionist, family-centred maternity care. By undermining the rationales for routine obstetrical practices, family physicians created a climate in which not performing unproven interventionist obstetrical practices was defensible. This was considered a necessary and useful tactic for securing and maintaining a share of the maternity care market.

Midwifery questioning of episiotomy: a postscript

In contrast to the earlier period when evidence-based episiotomy critiques rapidly accumulated within the nurse-midwifery literature, after 1987 the questioning of episiotomy began slowing. Between 1988 and 1995, eight more studies and one editorial appeared in the literature, primarily in the *Journal of Nurse-Midwifery*, undermining the medical rationales offered for performing routine episiotomy. The studies consisted of one non-randomized prospective study, five retrospective studies, one case control study and a meta-analysis. These studies provided evidence that episiotomy:

- was not related to improved perineal muscle function (Cosner *et al.*, 1991a) but was associated with urinary stress incontinence (Skoner *et al.*, 1994);
- did not prevented severe perineal lacerations (Röckner *et al.*, 1989);
- did not heal better than a spontaneous tear (McGuinness *et al.*, 1991); and

- avoiding the operation did not adversely affect maternal or fetal outcomes (Anderson & Greener, 1991).

Other studies examined factors associated with perineal outcome or episiotomy (Lydon-Rochelle *et al.*, 1995) or revealed that midwives performed fewer episiotomies compared with obstetricians (Kaufman & McDonald, 1988; Anonymous, 1993a; 1993b). Still others showed that the prenatal practice of perineal massage decreased the need for episiotomy and the incidence of perineal laceration (Avery & Van Arsdale, 1987). During these years there was also an editorial that questioned the value of episiotomy for shoulder dystocia, a widely accepted obstetrical indication for the operation (Piper & McDonald, 1994).

The challenging of episiotomy within obstetrics catches on: 1988–1995

In the USA and Canada the questioning of episiotomy in the obstetrical literature only began to take off toward the end of the 1980s. Between 1988 and 1995 there were four editorials or letters to the editor questioning the justification for routine episiotomy. Evidence against it produced by obstetricians began rapidly accumulating during these years as well. For example, a handful of review articles and more than a dozen retrospective or prospective studies failed to provide evidence for the presumed benefits of episiotomy. The questioning of the operation in the non-obstetrical and family practice literature also mounted during these years. To appreciate the extent to which routine episiotomy came under fire and the evidence against the practice rapidly accumulated during these years, it is useful to review briefly the obstetrical literature in chronological order.

In 1988 there were no episiotomy critiques in the obstetrical literature. In 1989, however, a retrospective study examining the relationship between both episiotomy and the use of stirrups for delivery and the occurrence of severe perineal lacerations was published in the *American Journal of Obstetrics and Gynecology* (Borgatta *et al.*, 1989). This study revealed that severe perineal lacerations were most likely when women were delivered with both an episiotomy and stirrups (28%) and least likely when neither episiotomy nor stirrups were used (0.9%). These researchers concluded that the selective use of episiotomy and stirrups minimized perineal trauma during spontaneous delivery.

Within two months, a lead article by Thorp and Bowes (1989) entitled 'Episiotomy: can its routine use be defended?' appeared in the 'Clinical Opinion' section of the *American Journal of Obstetrics and Gynecology*. This critique reviewed the literature for evidence that

routine episiotomy reduced perineal trauma and prevented subsequent pelvic relaxation. Thorp and Bowes (1989), finding little
empirical support for either of these claims, called for 'efforts ... [to] be
directed toward objectively ascertaining whether routine episiotomy is
truly beneficial' (p. 1030).

In the same issue of this journal, Wilcox *et al.*, from Johns Hopkins
University School of Public Health published a second report from
their retrospective matching study which focused on episiotomy and
its role in the incidence of perineal lacerations (Wilcox *et al.*, 1989). This
study found that the use of episiotomy was associated with a fourfold
increase in the incidence of severe lacerations. In a retrospective review
published in *Obstetrics and Gynecology*, its use was found to increase the
risk ninefold (Green & Soohoo, 1989).

It was also in this year that *Effective Care in Pregnancy and Childbirth*
(Chalmers *et al.*, 1989) and the paperback version *A Guide to Effective
Care in Pregnancy and Childbirth* (Enkin *et al.*, 1989) were released in the
USA and Canada with the recommendation that routine episiotomy be
abandoned.

In 1990, more retrospective studies indicating that midline episiotomy did not prevent severe perineal trauma continued appearing
in *Obstetrics and Gynecology* (Shiono *et al.*, 1990), and the *American
Journal of Obstetrics and Gynecology* (Combs *et al.*, 1990).

Still more evidence came in 1991 with the publication of a retrospective factor-searching study in *Obstetrics and Gynecology*. The study
by Walker *et al.* (1991) from the Department of Obstetrics and Gynecology at Mount Sinai Hospital in Toronto revealed that in their study
of nearly 9000 patients, the use of episiotomy was associated with a
fourfold increase in the likelihood of major perineal trauma. The claim
that episiotomy was prophylactic for pelvic floor relaxation was also
challenged in the obstetrical literature by nurse-midwives. Responding
to Thorp and Bowe's (1989) lead article, Cosner *et al.* (1991b) in a letter
to the editor of the *American Journal of Obstetrics and Gynecology*, presented the results of a longitudinal study which involved taking
multiple pelvic muscle measurements of 22 women who had given
birth vaginally without an episiotomy. They concluded that 'restitution
of the pelvic muscle may occur over time and therefore episiotomy for
prophylactic use in the prevention of pelvic muscle relaxation may not
be defensible' (p. 936). Thorp and Bowes (1991) replied by calling for
follow-up studies of the long-term effects of method of delivery.

In 1992, still more evidence that episiotomy was not prophylactic for
pelvic floor relaxation came from a paper reporting the results of a
Danish prospective non-randomized study in *Obsterics and Gynecology*.
The study, which examined symptoms of urinary stress incontinence
caused by pregnancy or delivery, found that mediolateral episiotomy
was associated with the development, not prevention, of stress

incontinence (Viktrup *et al.*, 1992). Around the same time, the claim that episiotomy prevented fetal injury was also challenged in a review in *Clinics in Perinatalogy* (Ahn *et al.*, 1992) which evaluated the preferred route of delivery for low birthweight infants. Further evidence that lower episiotomy rates did not compromise the infant or mother was published by Chambliss *et al.* (1992) in *Obstetrics and Gynecology*. This study, an RCT of midwifery and physician management of birth, found that women in the midwife-managed group had significantly fewer episiotomies and severe perineal lacerations. There was also no difference in neonatal outcome between the groups.

In 1993 one retrospective cohort study in *Obstetrics and Gynecology* revealed that in operative deliveries, midline episiotomy increased rather than decreased the risk of severe perineal laceration, and called for an RCT (Helwig *et al.*, 1993). Another smaller study revealed that women who had suffered rupture of the anal sphincter were six times more likely to report incontinence of flatus and, because of the direct relationship between median episiotomy and severe perineal laceration, the authors concluded 'it seems prudent to minimize the use of midline episiotomy' (Crawford *et al.*, 1993:530). A twenty-year retrospective study revealed that the incidence of episiotomy had declined during the study period and that the use of the operation was related to the use of epidurals (Farabow *et al.*, 1993).

Within obstetrics, the questioning of episiotomy which had the greatest impact by far during these years was by *Williams Obstetrics* (Cunningham *et al.*, 1993). For the first time since the tenth edition in 1950, this widely disseminated and respected textbook advised:

'... episiotomy should not be performed routinely. The procedure should be applied selectively for appropriate conditions ...' (Cunningham *et al.*, 1993: 389).

In 1994, two review articles were published, one in *Obstetrical and Gynecological Survey* and the other in *Clinical Obstetrics and Gynecology*. The former reviewed the obstetrical literature for the risks of dehiscence and rectovaginal fistula formation from episiotomy and concluded:

'overall, these studies do not indicate that elective episiotomy offers a clear benefit for delivery ... It is clearly evident that episitomy is a risk factor in the occurrence of third- and fourth-degree laceration and rectovaginal fistula formation. Hence, selective, rather than routine, use of episiotomy is preferable in the absence of risk factors for laceration ...' (Homsi *et al.*, 1994:807).

The latter review entitled, 'Episiotomy and early repair of dehiscence', while focusing more on episiotomy repair and complications, nevertheless disputed the presumed benefits of episiotomy and reported,

'...there appears to be little justification for routine performance of episiotomy' (Ramin & Gilstrap, 1994:816).

Also, Klein *et al.* (1994) published a post hoc secondary analysis of trial data in the *American Journal of Obstetrics and Gynecology* which showed once again that, contrary to traditional obstetrical belief, perineal and pelvic floor morbidity was greatest among women receiving a median episiotomy versus those remaining intact or sustaining a spontaneous tear.

During the late 1980s and early 1990s the questioning of episiotomy was also quite extensive in the non-obstetrical literature, in the general as well as family practice literature. For example, in 1987, the relationship between use of episiotomy and postpartum dyspareunia was once again highlighted in a review article in *Archives of Sexual Behavior* (Reamy & White, 1987). That same year, more evidence that episiotomy did not prevent severe perineal lacerations came from a study published in the *Canadian Medical Association Journal* which documented changes in obstetrical practices at one obstetrical unit in Oxford during a four-year period (1980–1984) (Reynolds & Yudkin, 1987). Analysis of nearly 25 000 births revealed that there had been a 28% decline in the use of episiotomy for primips and a 21% decrease in the use of episiotomy for multips with no corresponding increase in the rate of severe lacerations. This study provided evidence that the lowering of episiotomy rates was safe as well as feasible.

The following year, Klein, a family physician, published 'Rites of passage: episiotomy and the second stage of labour' (1988). Klein used this paper to make a plea for the reassessment of family physicians' management of the second stage and to increase awareness about the first North American RCT of episiotomy and the first ever RCT to evaluate the effectiveness of median episiotomy, which he and others in Montreal were in the process of carrying out.

In 1990, a group of family physicians called into question the presumed benefit of episiotomy preventing tears with a retrospective study investigating the relationship between maternal birthing position and perineal outcome. The study, published in the *Journal of Family Practice*, revealed that women giving birth in the lithotomy position were more likely to have an episiotomy or severe laceration than women giving birth in a birthing bed (Olson *et al.*, 1990).

Ensuring wide dissemination by publishing in the *Journal of the American Medical Association*, Banta and Thacker (1990), in a paper entitled 'The case for reassessment of health care technology. Once is not enough', presented the results of the Dublin and West Berkshire RCTs and Thorp and Bowes (1989) lead article in the *American Journal of Obstetrics and Gynecology* to emphasize the lack of evidence supporting the use of episiotomy.

The journal *Birth* also raised questions about the value of episiotomy with the publication of a prospective case controlled study of childbirth classes which showed that episiotomy was significantly associated with severe lacerations (Hetherington, 1990), and a commentary that offered arguments against episiotomy and in favour of squatting for birth (Paciornik, 1990). The publication of the results of a survey of obstetrical practitioners in *Social Science and Medicine* in 1990 provided insight for the first time into practitioners' attitudes and use of episiotomy. The study found that routine episiotomy was favoured by obstetricians, less by family physicians, even less by nurse-midwives and least by lay midwives (Graham *et al.*, 1990).

An important contribution to the challenging of episiotomy was made in the early 1990s by members of the Obstetrical Interest Group of the North American Primary Care Research Group (NAPCRG) with the publication of what are essentially evidence-based clinical practice guidelines about management of labour and delivery in the *Journal of Family Practice* (Smith *et al.*, 1991) and *American Family Physician* (Smith *et al.*, 1993). Specifically related to episiotomy, after critically reviewing the literature they recommended that 'a restrictive policy towards episiotomy should be adopted' (Smith *et al.*, 1993:1479).

In 1992, Klein *et al.* published the results of their RCT of episiotomy in the premier issue of the *Online Journal of Current Clinical Trials*, the first peer-reviewed medical journal distributed by computer (online). The trial compared the USA and Canadian practice of liberal use of episiotomy to avoid perineal tears with a policy of restricting the use of the operation to specific fetal and/or maternal indications. The trial found that restricting the use of episiotomy in primiparous women was associated with sutured perineal trauma similar to that of the routine approach. Multiparous women in the restricted episiotomy group, however, gave birth significantly more often with an intact perineum. Severe perineal lacerations were found to be associated with the use of median episiotomy. No differences were found between groups in terms of postpartum perineal pain, antepartum or three-month postpartum muscle strength, and urinary or pelvic floor symptoms. Finding no evidence that liberal or routine use of episiotomy prevents perineal trauma or pelvic floor relaxation, Klein *et al.* concluded, 'it is our recommendation that liberal or routine use of episiotomy be abandoned' (Klein *et al.*, 1992; paragraph 59).

The results of the Montreal trial (Klein *et al.*, 1992) were further disseminated when they became the source of both an editorial in the *Online Journal of Current Clinical Trials* entitled 'Episiotomy: to cut or not to cut?' (Kaufmann, 1992) and a commentary in the journal *Birth*, 'The final fatal blow to routine episiotomy' (Reynolds, 1993).

More questions were raised about the necessity and value of episiotomy by a descriptive study published in 1993 in the *Journal of the Louisiana State Medical Society*. This paper reported on nearly 1000 uncomplicated vaginal deliveries in Lucea, Jamaica which yielded 742 women (75%) who were discharged with intact perineums, 253 women (25%) who suffered a laceration of whom 172 (17.3%) required suturing, and only 3 women who received an episiotomy (Doherty & Cohen, 1993). By contrasting the very low use of episiotomy in Jamaica with the routine use of the operation in the USA, the authors questioned whether the use of episiotomy in the latter was excessive.

In 1995, for the first time in North America, two studies were published in the medical literature specifically about changing physicians' use of episiotomy. One paper presented the results of a before-and-after study which used a continuous quality improvement (CQI) programme to reduce episiotomy rates in one hospital (Reynolds, 1995). This study involved applying educational strategies to promote better understanding of what constitutes an appropriate episiotomy and true fetal distress as well as suggesting ways to reduce maternal exhaustion and manoeuvres to protect the perineum during childbirth. By the end of the study period (one year) the overall episiotomy rate had declined from 44.5% to 33.3%.

The other study by Klein *et al.* (1995) examined the beliefs and behaviours of the physicians who had participated in their RCT of episiotomy. They found that physicians' beliefs about episiotomy were strongly related to their use of episiotomy and other obstetrical procedures during the trial. Physicians with favourable attitudes toward episiotomy were less likely to randomize patients into the trial and more likely to justify exclusion of women from the trial on the grounds of 'fetal distress' or Caesarean section. Once a woman was entered in the trial, these physicians had greater difficulty limiting the use of episiotomy in the restricted arm of the trial. Furthermore, women in their care were more likely to receive oxytocin augmentation and to have shorter labours. This study formed the basis of a 1996 *Lancet* commentary on the influence of beliefs on clinicians' behaviour (Graham, 1996).

The studies by Reynolds and Klein *et al.* are both important because they signify acceptance of the need to reduce the use of episiotomy and the identification of barriers to changing physician behaviour.

Chapter 7

The Process of Change

This chapter focuses on the process of change in maternity care. It begins by contrasting the recent challenging of episiotomy in the USA with what occurred in the United Kingdom and suggests why this questioning may have had so much less impact in the USA than in the UK. The rest of the chapter summarizes my findings. The earlier chapters traced and analysed the evolution of episiotomy in chronological order; this highlights the most salient aspects of the change process: the factors and forces implicated in both the introduction of routine episiotomy and the challenging of prophylactic episiotomy during the 1970s and 80s.

The limited impact of the questioning of episiotomy in the USA

As has been shown, in a very short period of time in the UK, the lay and professional questioning of the practice of routine episiotomy sufficiently undermined the presumed rationale for the operation that some practitioners no longer felt compelled to perform the operation routinely. In addition, the questioning eventually led to the operation becoming so controversial within the expert medical community that the mounting of three RCTs (Harrison et al., 1984; Sleep et al., 1984; House et al., 1986) became justified. The results of these trials then provided evidence for the restricted use of episiotomy.

In the USA, the initial challenging of episiotomy failed to generate much controversy within obstetrics and did not generate national debate about the value of the operation. For example, Murray Enkin, a prominent Canadian obstetrician-researcher, was unable to secure outside funding for what would have been the first North American RCT of episiotomy in the early 1980s. Looking at the literature, had it not been for an editorial Enkin wrote about the experience in the journal *Birth. Issues in Perinatal Care and Education* (Enkin et al., 1984), there is virtually no indication that routine episiotomy was even being questioned by North American obstetricians in the early 1980s.

With obstetrical controversy about the routine use of episiotomy failing to materialize in the early 1980s and with obstetricians attending the vast majority of all deliveries in the USA (obstetricians deliver 80% of babies), it is hardly surprising the episiotomy rate in the USA did not decline. By comparing the questioning of episiotomy which took place in the USA with that which occurred in the UK during the same time period, a number of factors can be identified which help explain why the use of episiotomy only began to really drop toward the end of the 1980s.

First of all, the extent to which the practice of episiotomy had become obstetric orthodoxy differed greatly between the UK and USA. In the UK, the questioning of episiotomy occurred at the same time that the use of the operation was becoming routine. In the USA, the questioning occurred after the practice had already been routine for more than four decades. In other words, the routine use of episiotomy was considerably more established in American obstetrics, with a history and lore dating back to at least the 1940s, making the earliest challenging of the practice seem heretical. Furthermore, because episiotomy was so widely accepted and had been established for so long, obstetricians had difficulty even contemplating conducting a delivery without performing an episiotomy because of all the 'dangers' they had been taught were inherent in the birth process. In contrast, in the UK, many midwives and even obstetricians were more open to questioning the routine use of episiotomy because they often had some residual knowledge of successful experiences of delivering women without an episiotomy and severe perineal trauma.

Also in the USA there was no 'National Perinatal Epidemiology Unit' (NPEU) as there was in Oxford to promote the scientific evaluation of obstetrical and midwifery practices. The impact of Iain Chalmers and the NPEU on creating a climate more receptive to evidence-based practice should not be underestimated. Had this not been the case, Chalmers and his colleagues at the NPEU would not have been dubbed the Baader-Meinhof gang of obstetrics by a leading British obstetrician. In the USA there were no comparable individuals or group which provide this type of national direction and leadership on maternity care research issues.

Other factors relate to both who was doing the questioning and how they went about doing it. It must be remembered that in the UK the intense lay questioning of the operation was spearheaded by one extremely prominent and influential childbirth educator and reformer, Sheila Kitzinger. Kitzinger, with assistance from the NCT and AIMS, organized and directed a campaign against routine episiotomy. This campaign raised women's and health care professionals' consciousness about the unproven prophylactic benefits of episiotomy and the adverse effects associated with the operation, and produced a fertile ground on which RCTs of episiotomy could be undertaken. Although considerable lay questioning of episiotomy also took place in the USA, no one person of Kitzinger's stature took it upon themselves to mount and lead a crusade against the operation. As one key informant remarked about Kitzinger, 'Who else is able to organize a demonstration of 10 000 people at the drop of a hat?'.

The context in which the questioning of episiotomy came about was also different in America. In the UK, Kitzinger and other childbirth activists mobilized opposition to the routine use of episiotomy by focusing specifically on the operation and drawing attention to it as a separate or single issue independent of other childbirth practices. In the USA, the childbirth reform movement focused attention on the medicalization of the entire process of childbirth. Episiotomy was but one of many obstetrical procedures questioned. As Swenson of *Our Bodies, Ourselves* describes it:

'...the feminist perspective was already challenging medical authority, challenging male dominance, challenging sexism that we found inherent in virtually *every* medical encounter. And then by extension beginning to question everything that was done, of which birthing was only part. So glancingly, I say, the episiotomy was included in that list, but only so far as we were already questioning the positioning, we were questioning the anaesthesia, analgesia, we were questioning the exclusion of midwifery knowledge, the exclusion of homebirth' (interview with Norma Swenson).

At no time did the issue of routine episiotomy in the USA ever become an issue in and of itself as it had in the UK. With the exception of Kitzinger and Simkin's (1984; 1986) book, almost all the lay questioning of episiotomy was embedded in critiques about childbirth in the USA. Differing from the UK, no pressure groups like the NCT or AIMS took up the cause against routine episiotomy, no one surveyed women to elicit their experiences with the operation as Kitzinger had done, and there were no newspaper articles devoted solely to the issue of episiotomy. Compared with what appeared to be a concerted and organized campaign against routine episiotomy in the UK, the questioning of episiotomy in the USA lacked leadership, direction and intensity. As another key informant remarked:

'Well, the United States doesn't have a Sheila Kitzinger or a Beverley Beech. There isn't anybody in the United States with that kind of charisma. Sheila had a *lot* to do with the drop in the episiotomy rate in Britain, not she alone, but she and the women she mobilized. Doris [Haire] does not carry the kind of weight that Sheila does. Sheila knows the media. I think there just isn't anybody in the United States like Sheila. Doris has been a lobbyist. I mean, Doris has her American Foundation for Maternal Child Health and she does have a lot of influence, she is a lobbyist in Washington. But as far as procedures go, she hasn't the clout that Sheila has. And you've got Norma Swenson and her group [the Boston Women's Health Book Collective]. I think they carry a fair bit of weight. But once again I don't know how much. You've got David Stewart and the NAPSAC, you've got the ICEA, you've got ASPO [the American Society for Psychoprophylaxis in Obstetrics], none of them have really captured ... and you've got all sorts of splinter organizations that don't speak with one voice' (Anonymous).

The lay questioning of episiotomy also had less of an effect on American obstetricians because of the availability of alternative maternity options. Women most strongly opposed to routine episiotomy have increasingly chosen to avoid the operation by having their babies at home (Hazell, 1976; Maynard, 1977) or in birth centres (Davis, 1976; Norwood, 1978) with the assistance of lay and nurse-midwives. Instead of pursuing the issue about the use of episiotomy with obstetricians, many of these women have essentially opted out of the mainstream of maternity care. By voting with their feet, the opposition to episiotomy felt by American obstetricians has been considerably less than what it could have been. In the UK, rather than opting out, childbearing women adopted the strategy of trying to change the system by challenging midwives and physicians to justify their use of episiotomy.

Another important difference between the USA and UK has to do with the role of midwives in questioning episiotomy. Although nurse-midwives in the USA and midwives in the UK were a major source of the published episiotomy critiques, their impact was very different. As British midwives attend 75% of births, their questioning of episiotomy was sufficient to cause physicians to take notice. As has already been argued in Chapter 5, given the high percentage of maternity cases cared for by midwives in the UK, a reduction in the use of episiotomy by even a small number of midwives would have translated into an appreciable decline in the national episiotomy rate. In the USA, nurse-midwives attend less than 5% of births; for this reason, their episiotomy critiques have been easily ignored by the obstetrical community, and their avoidance of the operation would have had a negligible effect on the national episiotomy rate.

Focusing more on obstetrician related factors, with the exception of Edward Stewart Taylor, the editor of *Obstetrical and Gynecological Survey* (1982), the other obstetricians who were among the first to question episiotomy were not widely known authorities. This differed from the UK where several quite influential medical authorities added their voices to the questioning (e.g. Professors Morris and Russell, Iain Chalmers and Luke Zander).

At the same time, the obstetrical establishment and leading obstetrical authorities continued to openingly support routine episiotomy and promulgated the putative benefits of the operation. For example, *Williams Obstetrics*, the most popular obstetrical text in the USA advised obstetricians and medical students of the alleged benefits of episiotomy. The fifteenth through to the seventeenth editions of this textbook authoritatively stated the reasons for the popularity of the operation: it 'substitutes a straight, neat surgical incision for the ragged laceration that otherwise frequently results. It is easier to repair and heals better than a tear. With a mediolateral episiotomy, the likelihood of lacerations into the rectum is reduced' (Pritchard *et al.*, 1985:347–8). As has already been noted, the sixteenth and seventeenth editions of *Williams Obstetrics* respectively acknowledged the questioning of the advantages of episiotomy by Cogan and Edmunds (1977) and then by Thacker and Banta (1983). In both cases, however, this questioning was then dismissed with only the observation that the frequency of gynaecological problems has decreased since births have taken place in hospital with episiotomy.

Furthermore, well-respected obstetricians such as David Danforth (1974) and J.R. Wilson (1984), along with others such as Robert Bradley (1981), the author of *Husband-coached Childbirth*, and Clark Gillespie (1992), Fellow of both the American College of Obstetricians and Gynecologists and the Royal College of Obstetricians and Gynaecologists (London), continued to strongly endorse the use of routine episiotomy and advised women of the wonderful 'benefits' of the operation.

The writings of these obstetricians and other episiotomy enthusiasts also reveal two other factors that suppressed obstetricians' willingness to consider questioning episiotomy. One was the almost fanatical belief in the alleged benefits of episiotomy. Obstetricians simply took for granted the claims of benefit made for episiotomy and were therefore not prepared to entertain any notion that their faith in episiotomy might be misplaced. For example, a 1976 national survey of 249 certified obstetricians (Lake, 1976) revealed that close to half reported 'always' performing episiotomy. Practically all agreed that episiotomy prevents perineal tearing, three-quarters said it also protects the infant's head from trauma, and more than one-third were more strongly in favour of episiotomy than they had been five years earlier.

Likewise, many obstetricians also held strongly to the belief that the operation benefited both the mother and her spouse sexually. While this alleged benefit of episiotomy is often not made explicitly in the literature, it is often mentioned by obstetricians in private as an important reason for performing the operation. The following passage by Gideon Panter, MD, a diplomat of the ABOG, is probably representative of the view of many obstetricians in the early 1980s. In an article for expectant mothers in *Parents* magazine, Panter remarked about episiotomy:

'I explain to my patients that, for the most part, episiotomy is performed solely to help preserve the strength of their vaginal muscles, which can be a factor in maintaining a good sexual relationship in the future. Physical changes occur as men age, and considerably more direct stimulation is often needed if an older man is to maintain an erection... An episiotomy, then, is better described as being done as much for the husband's sake in later life as it is for the wife's benefit' (Panter, 1980:88).

Another more psychological reason obstetricians were unwilling to reconsider their use of episiotomy had to do with their feeling that the profession was under attack. Many obstetricians were angered that they and their professional judgment and autonomy were being questioned. This resentment, along with their strong beliefs in the value of episiotomy, led them to simply dismiss or ignore the questioning instead of grappling with it, as occurred in the UK. The following passage from Gillespie's book *Your Pregnancy Month by Month*, which has sold over 150 000 copies, exemplifies the mood of the time. Note the condescending and disparaging tone directed at the 'cultists' and 'extremists' doing the questioning and Gillespie's unswerving allegiance to the alleged prophylactic benefits of episiotomy.

'Although your episiotomy may cause you some discomfort after you deliver, it heals much better than a tear and gives you much better support for later years... Lately the episiotomy, as with so many other important things, has fallen victim to the frantic race among some of the cultists to get motherhood back to nature before things get too good. Many women who do not receive interventions such as a deep and proper episiotomy tend to develop several specific disorders from the resultant muscle and skin damage. The rectum and the bladder tend to push through the damaged muscle support and bulge into the vagina, causing conditions known as rectocele (from the rectum) and cystocele (from the bladder), which require surgical intervention somewhere along the line. Relaxation of the vagina can also lead to a loss of sexual sensation. This loss of sexual sensation is felt (or not felt) by both partners. The extremists of the "natural" movement ignore this problem and state that psychogenic stimulation outside the vagina compensates for this loss of vaginal sensation, which is exactly the same as saying smelling ice cream is as good as eating it' (Gillespie, 1992:226,227).

Why the declining use of episiotomy during the late 1980s?

Starting in 1988, the national episiotomy rate began declining and within six years had gone from 59% to 50.4%, an absolute and relative decline of 9% and 15% respectively. What accounts for this turning point? While there can be little doubt that *Effective Care in Pregnancy and Childbirth* (Chalmers *et al.*, 1989) and *A Guide to Effective Care in Pregnancy and Childbirth* (Enkin *et al.*, 1989) systematically reviewed and summarized the best research evidence available to show that routine episiotomy was not beneficial, it would seem that neither of these books had an immediate or very large impact on obstetrical practices in the USA during the first few years following publication. By April 1991, only 450 copies of *ECPC* and 1000 copies of the *Guide* had been sold in the USA, suggesting that few clinicians had ready access to them (Sisk, 1993:481).

On the other hand, the mounting episiotomy critiques, written primarily by obstetricians toward the end of the 1980s, were finding their way into the textbooks. In the eighteenth edition of *Williams Obstetrics* published in 1989, the following paragraph was added which reveals that the questioning of episiotomy was successfully raising doubts about the taken-for-granted presumed benefits of the operation.

'More recently, the advantages provided by episiotomy have been questioned by some individuals (Thacker & Banta, 1983). One commonly cited but unproven benefit of routine episiotomy is that it prevents pelvic relaxation – that is, cystocele, rectocele, and urinary incontinence. Obviously, if the perineal incision is made at the time of maximal distention, then this benefit might be limited. Gass and colleagues (1986), as well as Thorp and co-workers (1987), recommend that routine episiotomy be re-evaluated since it possibly was associated with an increased incidence of anal sphincter and rectal tears. Reynolds and Yudkin (1987) studied nearly 25 000 deliveries at the John Radcliffe Hospital in Oxford, and reported that the episiotomy rate in nulliparas decreased from 73% in 1980 to 45% in 1984. During this same time, the incidence of second-degree tears increased from 7 to 20 per 1000, but the incidence of third-degree lacerations was unchanged at about 5 per 1000' (Cunningham *et al.*, 1989:323).

As the following passages reveal, the subsequent edition of *Williams Obstetrics* (1993) incorporated many more of the evidence-based episiotomy critiques, indicating that these critiques were responsible for overturning the textbook's decades' old position on routine episiotomy.

'...it is easier to repair, but the long-held beliefs that postoperative pain is less and healing is improved with an episiotomy compared to a tear appear not to be true (Larsson and colleagues, 1991)...
The advantages provided by an episiotomy have been questioned by some individuals (Borgatta, 1989; Larsson, 1991; Sleep, 1984; Thacker and Banta, 1983; Thorp, 1987, 1989; Viktrup, 1992; Wilcox, 1989; and all their co-workers). One commonly cited but unproven benefit of routine episiotomy is that it prevents pelvic relaxation, that is, cystocele, rectocele, and urinary incontinence. Obviously, if the perineal incision is made at the time of maximal distention, then this benefit might be limited. Borgatta (1989), Gass (1986), Thorp (1987, 1989), Wilcox (1989), and their co-workers maintain that routine episiotomy is associated with an increased incidence of anal sphincter and rectal tears. Reynolds and Yudkin (1987) studied nearly 25 000

deliveries at the John Radcliffe Hospital in Oxford, and reported that the episiotomy rate in nulliparas decreased from 73% in 1980 to 45% in 1984....' (Cunningham *et al.*, 1993:389).

While national episiotomy statistics from 1994 onward are still not available, it will be interesting to see if the episiotomy rate continues to decline and by how much during the mid 1990s. Should there be a noticeable drop in the episiotomy rate after 1993, the Montreal episiotomy RCT (Klein *et al.*, 1992) may be able to take much of the credit for it. Although the study did not receive a great deal of attention in the medical literature, perhaps because it was published in the first issue of *Online Journal of Current Clinical Trials*, it did receive considerable publicity in the print and electronic media. For example, articles about the study appeared in *The Washington Post, The Washington Times, The Boston Globe, The New York Times, The Los Angeles Times, The Baltimore Sun, The Atlanta Journal, The Philadelphia Inquirer, USA Today* and *The Reader's Digest*. No doubt many maternity care providers would have seen or heard about the study results in the popular press. Perhaps more importantly, given the force women can exert on maternity care providers, literally millions of present and future childbearing women would have also read the trial results with interest and discussed them with their maternity care providers.

Summary of the routinization of episiotomy

Agents responsible

This research demonstrates how identifiable individuals championing a particular cause (i.e. engaging in claims-making activities) can bring about innovation in maternity care. In the USA, the routinization of episiotomy can be traced to two groups of obstetrician/gynaecologists who lobbied for the operation between 1915 and 1935.

The first group consisted of a handful of prominent American obstetrician/gynaecologists. Between 1915 and 1925, these physicians lobbied their equally distinguished colleagues at national meetings of the two elite obstetric and gynaecology societies to perform elective episiotomy. As part of their pleas for the prophylactic performance of episiotomy, they claimed that the operation prevented perineal lacerations, returned the perineum to its prepregnancy state, and shortened labour thereby reducing or preventing infant mortality and morbidity. They also emphasized their strong belief that if performed prophylactically, episiotomy would prevent future gynaecological problems that develop decades after childbirth. These pleas received considerable exposure when they were later published in leading obstetrical journals.

Between 1925 and 1935, a somewhat larger group of American episiotomy protagonists echoed the same claims, but in addition declared
that every, or nearly every, first-time mother would benefit from the
operation. Although these episiotomy protagonists were specialists in
obstetrics and gynaecology, they were not among the elite of the profession. Reflecting their less prominent stature, they tended to make
their pleas for the routine or indiscriminate use of episiotomy at local
obstetrical association meetings and in national or local obstetric
journals.

That there was an absence of scientific evidence for the claims being
made underscores the effectiveness of the championing of routine
episiotomy by particular obstetricians. None of the benefits claimed for
episiotomy were evidence-based. Therefore the subsequent adoption
of routine episiotomy by American physicians suggests the greater
influence of the claims-makers and their claims rather than scientific
research.

In the UK, the routinization of episiotomy in the mid 1960s and 1970s
came about quite differently. There, the liberal use of episiotomy
occurred without any overt lobbying by particular obstetricians. This is
not to say, however, that British consultant obstetricians did not in any
way influence the greater use of episiotomy. While individual obstetricians may not have publicly campaigned for the greater use of episiotomy, collectively they exerted direct and indirect pressure on
midwives and physicians working in their maternity units to use the
operation more frequently.

Factors encouraging the adoption of routine episiotomy

This research has identified three factors common to both the USA and
UK that facilitated the routine use of episiotomy in these countries.
These factors fall into three broad categories:

- changes in the dominant belief system within obstetrics;
- changes in maternity care practices; and
- changes taking place within the obstetric and midwifery
  professions.

In the USA, the acceptance of routine episiotomy had to do with a
shift in the conceptualization of the nature of childbirth. As long as the
obstetrical belief system held that childbirth was a normal process,
physicians considered routine surgical intervention highly unnecessary and inappropriate. In the 1800s, the strong acceptance of the belief
that childbirth and the functioning of the perineum was a normal
physiological process discouraged acceptance of the pleas of the

nineteenth-century episiotomy enthusiasts. During the 1920s and 1930s childbirth was recast as a pathogenic and pathological process. Once the obstetrical belief system supported the view of childbirth as abnormal, prophylactic intervention believed to minimize or prevent this pathology became not only acceptable to physicians but also desirable. In other words, the advocacy of routine episiotomy became compatible with the belief system within obstetrics.

The argument can also be made that changes in the British obstetrical belief system indirectly encouraged the liberal use of episiotomy during the 1970s. Although British obstetricians continued to believe that childbirth was largely a normal process most appropriately cared for by midwives, during the 1970s the practices of induction and 'active management of labour' became increasingly accepted. The philosophy behind these approaches was that obstetrical intervention (induction and augmentation) could effectively and safely improve upon the physiological process of childbirth. This new belief in the superiority of obstetrical intervention was compatible with, and smoothed the way for, a more liberal use of episiotomy.

Changes in maternity practices affected the use of episiotomy in several ways. In both the US and UK, the shifting of place of birth from home to hospital coincided with the increased use of episiotomy. As the proportion of women giving birth in hospital increased, practical impediments to performing the operation decreased. In contrast to the conditions found at homebirths, the use of episiotomy was facilitated in hospital by ready availability of the facilities and technology necessary to safely carry out the procedure. This included such things as aseptic operating room conditions, proper lighting, anaesthesia and capable assistants. With the integration of British midwives into hospitals in the 1970s, their use of episiotomy was also encouraged because of the availability of medical practitioners found in the hospital. Because the law required episiotomies cut by British midwives to be repaired by a physician, midwives attending homebirths were reluctant to perform the operation because of the inconvenience of having to wait for a physician to arrive to suture the incision. In hospital, this barrier to the midwifery use of episiotomy was removed, or perceived by midwives to be removed.

The nearly one-hundred per cent hospitalization of birthing women also encouraged the increased use of episiotomy for reasons of birth attendant convenience. Unlike a homebirth where there is only one labouring woman to attend at a time, in hospital physicians and midwives often find themselves caring for many labouring women simultaneously. Some of the increased use of episiotomy resulted from efforts to streamline the care of childbearing women in an attempt to deal with pressures generated by high patient volume found in hospitals. Birth attendants adopted the procedure because they believed that the operation shortened the second stage of labour, diminished the unpredictability of a perineal laceration, and was easier and quicker to repair than a spontaneous tear. From this perspective, pressures of the hospital environment coupled with birth attendants' perceptions that the operation expedited their work encouraged its use.

The phenomenon known as the cascade of intervention was also implicated in the initial increased use of episiotomy in both the USA and UK. This phenomenon refers to the situation whereby one particular intervention necessitates or encourages further interventions to facilitate or counteract the effects of the initial action. In the USA the growing use of forceps and obstetrical anaesthesia from the 1920s through the 1970s motivated the routine use of episiotomy. In the UK in the 1970s, the increasing use of induction had a similar effect. The rising use of forceps and induction in both countries coincided with the hospitalization of childbirth. It is important to note that the role of the cascade of intervention effect in increasing the use of episiotomy was limited to the initial rise in episiotomy use. In both countries, the routine episiotomy persisted after the use of forceps in the USA and induction in the UK declined in the 1970s, confirming that other factors were involved in maintaining the routine use of the operation.

The third category of factors common to the routinization of episiotomy in the USA and UK related to occupational transformations which occurred in American obstetrics during the 1920s through to the 1940s and in British midwifery during the 1970s. In the USA, this period can be characterized as a time of professional establishment. During these years, the obstetric profession struggled with self-definition and boundary setting. It was at this time that the obstetrical profession redefined itself and became the 'new obstetrics'. Obstetrics and gynaecology became formally united as one specialty, the nature of childbirth was recast from a normal or physiological process to a pathological one, and the approach of 'watchful expectancy' was replaced by an interventionist or activist ideology.

These changes, which were part of the transformation of the American obstetrical profession during the first half of the twentieth century, supported the increased use of episiotomy. At a philosophical level, prophylactic episiotomy appealed to physicians because its use symbolized acceptance of the new surgical obstetrics and rejection of the 'old' conservative or moderate school of obstetric thought. By performing prophylactic episiotomy the new obstetrician/gynaecologists distinguished themselves from 'old-fashioned midwifery'. It allowed them to claim that their methods had more to offer than those of the generalists and midwives. At the same time, prophylactic episiotomy was also stimulated because it appealed to obstetrician/gynaecologists' surgical aspirations. Surgical skill was now considered a defining characteristic of the profession.

Where the routinization of episiotomy in the USA resulted from efforts to elevate the status of the obstetric profession, it was reduction in the professional autonomy of midwives that prompted the increased use of episiotomy in the UK. During the 1970s, British domiciliary midwives were incorporated into hospitals with the move to hospitalize all births. At homebirths, midwives accepted total responsibility for the women they attended and called for medical assistance when they deemed it necessary. In hospital, midwives came under the direct supervision of consultant obstetricians. This shift in place of birth resulted in a dramatic reduction in the freedom of midwives to exercise clinical judgment. Midwifery use of episiotomy increased as consultant obstetricians influenced midwifery practice by setting formal and informal maternity unit policies and protocols about when and under what conditions midwives were to perform the operation.

Barriers to the routinization of episiotomy

This book has also identified a number of barriers to the routinization of episiotomy. In the USA, many of these barriers may be attributed to the notion that the period was simply not ripe for the greater use of episiotomy. In time, these barriers actually became factors that facilitated the routinization of episiotomy. In the 1800s, episiotomy enthusiasts were unsuccessful at encouraging the greater use of episiotomy because there was no theoretical justification for what they were proposing. Their pleas for episiotomy ran counter to the then prevalent obstetrical belief system that birth was a normal process that should not be interfered with unnecessarily. While congruence between proposed innovation and the existing belief system may facilitate change as described above, incongruence may effectively impede it.

Another factor that hindered the adoption of episiotomy in the 1800s but encouraged its use in the twentieth century was the availability of the technology necessary to carry out the operation safely. In the 1800s, nearly all births took place at home and limitations in medical technology, such as the lack of aseptic technique, underdeveloped suturing technology, poor lighting, untrained assistants, and inadequate local anaesthesia, discouraged the use of episiotomy. The availability of this technology eventually encouraged the use of episiotomy when it became readily available in the 1920s and 1930s.

The example of the efforts of the nineteenth-century episiotomy enthusiasts also revealed that the prominence and reputations of those involved in claims-making activities can influence the innovation process. In this case, the nineteenth-century episiotomy advocates lacked sufficiently prominent reputations to be able to neutralize the weighty pronouncements of the leading obstetrical authorities of the day who advised against using episiotomy. One other barrier to innovation identified by this example was consumer preference or perceived consumer preference. Nineteenth-century physicians, probably because they still perceived their position in the maternity care marketplace to be quite tenuous, were reluctant to ignore women's preferences not to receive an episiotomy.

Restrictive use of episiotomy in the UK prior to the mid 1960s also tells us something about barriers to innovation. In the UK, midwives attended the vast majority of births (many at home) and until 1967 were legally prohibited from performing the operation. In addition to the legal prohibition against the midwifery use of the operation, the liberal use of episiotomy was also discouraged by the obstetrical and midwifery belief system. Both midwives and physicians believed birth to be an essentially normal process with midwives being the appropriate birth attendants of normal births and obstetricians of abnormal births. This belief system discouraged the use of episiotomy as obstetricians saw no theoretical justification for allowing/encouraging midwives to surgically complicate a normal process.

The questioning and overturning of routine episiotomy

Agents responsible for the questioning of episiotomy

In contrast to individuals who were responsible for the routinization of episiotomy, agents challenging this practice were considerably more diverse. For example, in the UK, pressure from outside the professions of medicine and midwifery was responsible for initiating a debate about the value and benefit of routine episiotomy. This pressure originated from an anti-episiotomy campaign launched in the early 1970s by the UK's most prominent and influential childbirth educator and activist (Sheila Kitzinger). The campaign was bolstered by support from two national childbirth organizations (the NCT and AIMS) and many childbearing women. The lay challenge of episiotomy involved disputing the medical claims about the prophylactic benefits of episiotomy. This was done by surveying women about their experiences of episiotomy or by presenting the experiences of particular women, showing the serious and sometimes debilitating side-effects of episiotomy. These data were then used to publicly challenge clinicians to either prove that episiotomy was beneficial or stop performing it. By questioning episiotomy in the media in this way, those campaigning against the operation effectively transformed episiotomy into a social issue which was difficult for professionals to ignore.

Largely in response to the anti-episiotomy campaign and the questions that were being raised about the benefits of episiotomy, a few midwives began producing critiques of the practice in the early 1980s. Very shortly thereafter, midwifery questioning of episiotomy was eclipsed by criticism of the operation in the medical community. The initial professional episiotomy critiques were largely non-evidence-based and involved questioning the rationale for performing the operation. The effect of these critiques, however, was to generate uncertainty about the alleged benefits of the operation. Professional controversy about the operation intensified when episiotomy enthusiasts responded to critiques of the operation. By 1982, uncertainty about the value of episiotomy had become so great in the medical and midwifery communities that the mounting of RCTs became ethically justified and necessary to resolve the controversy. There was a state of clinical equipoise. Clinical equipoise is defined as a state of genuine uncertainty among the expert medical community regarding the comparative therapeutic merits of two alternative therapies resulting from present or imminent controversy over the preferred treatment (Freedman, 1987:141). The RCTs revealed that the routine use of episiotomy was indefensible and formed the basis of strong evidence-based episiotomy critiques.

During the 1980s the English national episiotomy rate declined substantially. Since much of this decline occurred prior to the publication of the results of the episiotomy RCTs and other evidence-based critiques, the lay anti-episiotomy campaign must be credited with prompting the reduction.

In the USA, the agents of change attempting to bring about a reduction in the use of episiotomy were quite similar to those found in the UK. However, the questioning of episiotomy persisted over a longer period of time and had considerably less impact on the national episiotomy rate. Again, pressure from outside of American medicine and nurse-midwifery precipitated the professional questioning of episiotomy. During the early and mid 1970s, prominent childbirth reformers and activists such as Doris Haire and Susanne Arms, along with the women's health movement and childbearing women, criticized routine episiotomy. This involved challenging the benefits claimed of episiotomy, thereby introducing uncertainty about the obstetric rationale for performing the operation. This lay questioning of episiotomy generated sufficient uncertainty about the value of episiotomy that some sympathetic professionals felt justified to investigate these lay criticisms and produce critiques for their own professional colleagues.

Of the professionals, nurse-midwives were the first to respond to the lay questioning of episiotomy in the late 1970s. Differing from the British midwifery critics of episiotomy, the majority of American nurse-midwife critiques were evidence-based. Typically using data from retrospective observational studies, these nurse-midwives refuted the medical rationale for performing the operation or demonstrated that the avoidance of episiotomy did not compromise the health of the mother or infant.

American medical questioning of episiotomy, in contrast to that in the UK, was very slow to develop and intensify. The first physicians to criticize episiotomy were family physicians in the early 1980s. Critiques of episiotomy by obstetricians did not appear until the mid 1980s. Most of the critiques written by American physicians were evidence-based, the majority presenting data challenging the belief that episiotomy prevents perineal trauma. Despite the greater proportion of evidence-based critiques in the USA, the questioning of episiotomy did not have a major impact on the medical community. In fact, unlike the UK, the episiotomy critiques of the early 1980s failed to produce sufficient uncertainty or clinical equipoise about the operation within the American medical community to encourage anyone to successfully mount an RCT to conclusively evaluate the alleged benefits of episiotomy.

Factors encouraging the questioning of routine episiotomy

An important factor that encouraged the questioning of episiotomy by professional critics had to do with resistance to obstetrical control and the staking out of turf or boundary setting. In both the UK and USA, midwifery interest in questioning episiotomy and the receptivity of rank-and-file midwives to this questioning related to concerns about professional preservation. In the UK, midwives seized on the episiotomy issue as a means of resisting obstetrical intrusion into midwifery practice and decision making. By the late 1970s and early 1980s, British midwives had come to the realization that by uncritically adopting some obstetric technologies such as routine episiotomy, they had surrendered to obstetricians much of their decision making autonomy as independent practitioners. They also realized that in performing routine episiotomy, the traditional and revered midwifery skill of managing the perineum so as to minimize perineal trauma was being lost, perhaps forever, if something was not done to prevent this. Midwives used the questioning of episiotomy to reassert the professional independence of midwifery decision making and to reclaim one of the hallmark skills of midwifery – delivery over an intact perineum.

In the USA, the questioning of episiotomy by nurse-midwives and family practitioners was strongly motivated by desires of these professional groups to secure their position in the delivery of maternity care. After being virtually abolished early in the century, the late 1970s was a time when American nurse-midwives were in the throes of restoring their profession as a legitimate provider of maternity care.

Nurse-midwives considered guarding the perineum as a hallmark of their profession, differentiating nurse-midwifery from obstetrical care. However, because of their tenuous position as a new profession they were extremely sensitive to exposing nurse-midwifery practices to medical criticism. To justify deviating from the obstetrical norm of routine episiotomy, nurse-midwives began developing a scientific body of nurse-midwifery knowledge to justify their non-interventionist practices. The evidence-based nurse-midwifery episiotomy critiques provided some of this empirical knowledge by showing it was not unsafe to avoid performing episiotomies as had been claimed by American obstetricians.

Similar to nurse-midwifery, during the 1970s, the specialty of family practice was also struggling to establish itself as a legitimate provider of maternity care. For this new developing specialty group, the questioning of episiotomy was part of an effort to stake claim to low risk, non-interventionist, family-centred maternity care. By using episiotomy critiques to undermine the obstetric rationale for routine episiotomy, family practitioners sought to justify their alternative form of maternity care.

Barriers to overturning routine episiotomy

By comparing and contrasting the questioning of episiotomy that took place in the UK with the USA, I have identified several reasons for the differential decline in the use of the operation in these countries. Most of the difference can be explained by who was doing the questioning and how they went about doing it. In the USA, significant obstetrical interest in questioning the practice never developed as it had in the UK. Within the American obstetrical community, the obstetricians who questioned the practice were too few in number and lacked the prominence necessary to seriously shake the profession's four-decade-old taken-for-granted acceptance of episiotomy. In other words, the obstetrical critics of episiotomy were unable to generate controversy or a debate about the procedure to counteract the well-respected obstetricians who continued to promote episiotomy. In addition to the insufficient obstetrical questioning of episiotomy, lay questioning of episiotomy in the USA also fell short compared with the situation in the UK.

While there was considerable lay criticism of episiotomy in the USA, an anti-episiotomy campaign never fully developed. For the most part, the lay critiques of episiotomy were embedded in criticisms of the medicalization of childbirth, a much broader issue. Episiotomy was discussed in the context of obstetrical intervention in general and was never made a separate issue as it was in the UK. Perhaps most importantly, in the USA, no one with the charisma and influence of Sheila Kitzinger organized and led the crusade against episiotomy. Furthermore, the questioning of episiotomy in the USA was not supported by national childbirth pressure groups. Because the lay questioning of episiotomy in the USA lacked focus, leadership and intensity it had less impact on American obstetricians.

Discussion

What generalizations does this case study allow us to make about the process of change in health care professions? This book has identified a number of determinants of change. Some are common to both the introduction of routine episiotomy and the overturning of this practice. Others are specific to one or the other phase in episiotomy use. The factors and forces which explain the evolution of episiotomy are advocacy and claims-making activity of specific individuals, the belief system, professional concerns, and an assortment of situation-specific factors. There is one other factor that deserves comment because of its apparently negligible role in either the acceptance or initial rejection of episiotomy. This factor is scientific evidence.

Advocacy and claims-making activity

This case study demonstrates that the forceful championing of an idea or practice by an influential individual or individuals can produce change. The process of advocating change involves making claims about the particular change being proposed. For example, the advocates of routine episiotomy claimed that the operation prevented perineal lacerations, infant morbidity and mortality, and future gynaecological problems. The anti-episiotomy advocates issued counter-claims disputing these alleged benefits of episiotomy.

Part of the success of this sort of advocacy results from the content of the claims being made. However, the success of claims-making activity is also strongly related to the stature and authority of those making claims. For example, the advocacy of episiotomy by the influential and authoritative Drs DeLee and Pomeroy is credited with increasing the use of episiotomy in the USA during the 1920s and 1930s. The pronouncements of authorities against a proposed change can also inhibit innovation. The obstetrical authorities of the late 1800s who opposed the nineteenth-century episiotomy enthusiasts discouraged the more frequent use of episiotomy. This example also suggests that authoritative change agents are more likely to be successful than change agents who lack prominent reputations.

The importance of the individual in championing change was also evident in the questioning of episiotomy that took place in the 1970s and 1980s. In the UK, advocacy against the liberal use of episiotomy by Sheila Kitzinger, the country's most influential childbirth activist, resulted in the declining use of episiotomy during the 1980s. This is in contrast to the US where no universally respected lay activist argued against episiotomy, and the rate has shown less of a decline.

While claims-making activity by prominent individuals can be an important and effective source of change, this research also shows that claims-making is not the only means by which changes in practice occur. In some cases, change can occur without the advocacy of identifiable individuals. In the UK during the 1970s, the liberal use of episiotomy developed without any overt lobbying for it.

The belief system

This book reveals that the prevailing belief system and accepted views of appropriate practice can greatly influence the acceptance of new ideas. For example, in the late 1800s, while American episiotomy enthusiasts issued pleas for the greater use of episiotomy, these pleas were rejected. The operation went against the prevailing theory that birth and the functioning of the perineum were usually physiological or normal processes not requiring surgical intervention. In the 1930s, the acceptance of routine episiotomy was greatly facilitated by the prevailing belief system which now held that birth was pathogenic. Obstetrical intervention was now thought to be required to safely negotiate a pathological process.

Professional concerns

In both the USA and UK factors relating to professional concerns influenced both the routinization and overturning of episiotomy. In the USA, efforts to redefine the mission of obstetrics as a surgical specialty ensured that obstetricians were receptive to the concept of routine episiotomy. In the UK, resistance to obstetrical intrusion into midwifery practice and the interests of midwives in preserving the profession's autonomy in clinical decision-making encouraged the restrictive use of episiotomy. In the USA, nurse-midwives' and family practitioners' questioning of routine episiotomy was encouraged by their concerns about establishing and maintaining their roles in maternity care and their desire to justify the avoidance of performing the episiotomy routinely. These examples show that when change serves the vested interests of a professional group (in addition to the perceived interests of consumers or patients) such change may be more readily accepted.

Situation-specific factors

This book also identifies a number of factors that encouraged either the acceptance of routine episiotomy or its decline. Routine episiotomy in both the USA and UK was greatly facilitated when the technology necessary to safely carry out the procedure became widely available. Similarly, technological developments increased the use of episiotomy as a by-product of other procedures. The increasing popularity of forceps and anaesthesia in the USA and induction in the UK necessitated the increased use of episiotomy because of the cascade of intervention effect.

A force that was not involved in the routinization of episiotomy but was central to the questioning of the practice is consumer pressure. In both the UK and USA, consumer critiques of episiotomy produced sufficient controversy to prompt some professionals to also question the practice. In some cases, childbirth activists personally influenced professionals to produce evidence-based critiques of routine episiotomy. From this example, it is seen that consumer pressure can be an extremely effective means of bringing about change in health care.

Scientific evidence

A factor that was consistently absent in both the acceptance and initial rejection of episiotomy was evidence. The routinization of episiotomy in the USA in the 1930s and 1940s and in the UK in the 1970s occurred without evidence that episiotomy was beneficial or safe. All of the claims made for episiotomy were unproven, yet the operation became widely accepted. As for the overturning of episiotomy, this too came about with minimal evidence that episiotomy was unnecessary. In the UK the results from RCTs showing that avoidance of episiotomy was no more harmful than performing episiotomy appeared only after the episiotomy rate had declined substantially. This indicates that lay questioning of episiotomy and controversy about the operation were more important in bringing about change than any evidence showing it was unnecessary.

While scientific evidence had little to do with the initial decline in the use of episiotomy, the evidence that was eventually produced showing routine episiotomy was not beneficial was very important as it was used by childbirth activists and professionals to justify the restricted use of episiotomy.

Some thoughts on studying change

The approach I adopted to study episiotomy blends aspects of the natural history, interactive and belief system approaches to study the process of change. The results of this research suggest that this integrative approach improves understanding of the determinants of change.

A major advantage of this model is that by focusing on the processionary and unfolding nature of change, it directs attention toward both successful and unsuccessful innovation. This permits insights to be drawn from the cases of failed attempts to bring about change as well as from cases of successful change. Applying McKinlay's (1981) natural history model of the career of a medical innovation to episiotomy would have provided a distorted view of the change process. McKinlay's seven stage career model does not consider failed attempts at bringing about change. By examining the unsuccessful efforts of the nineteenth-century episiotomy enthusiasts, the integrative model provides valuable clues about several of the determinants of change.

As suggested by the interactive model, change is a social activity and process. Thus, identifying the individuals and communities responsible for change as well as their ideas and interests is an effective strategy for maintaining a focus when tracing the evolution of change. Identifying claims-makers is a useful starting point. By constantly asking, 'What are they saying?', 'Who are they?', and 'What is their interest in this?', the process of putting the pieces of the innovation puzzle together is made much easier. Another lesson this approach teaches is to be as inclusive as possible in the analysis and to search out all the communities involved in producing change. For example, restricting attention to the professional literature would not have revealed the extent to which the overturning of episiotomy resulted from lay efforts.

One caveat, however, is that it is also important to keep in mind that some changes occur without overt lobbying efforts. This is why it is so essential to first trace and describe all changes or attempted changes chronologically, rather than focusing exclusively on discrete points in time when lobbying activities were successful and therefore appear to predominate.

Lastly, considering the prevailing belief system and its compatibility with the change being proposed can provide insight into the change process being investigated. However, using only a belief system approach to analyse the process of change might cause other important factors in the innovation process to be overlooked. For instance, how a change relates to practical issues such as existing technology may have little or nothing to do with the belief system in place.

Chapter 8

How to Challenge Obstetric Interventions

Ian D. Graham and Barbara Davies

This chapter suggests ways to challenge obstetric interventions and bring about change in maternity care. Although written specifically with individual midwifery practitioners in mind, the suggestions offered apply equally well to groups of practitioners, be they at the local, regional or national level, as well as managers and policy makers. These ideas may also be useful to other health care practitioners such as obstetric nurses, general practitioners and family physicians, obstetricians and antenatal educators.

In keeping with the theme of the book, this chapter is structured in terms of questions and actions that might be useful for health care practitioners considering challenging obstetric interventions. These questions and actions should be seen as a flexible guide (with suggestions) rather than a prescriptive list of steps. As the history of episiotomy shows change can be brought about in many different ways.

Most practitioners intend to provide the best care possible for their clients, but what is the best care? Do you ever wonder whether aspects of health care you provide are:

- necessary?
- safe?
- based on the latest scientific evidence?

Do you ever wonder whether the care you provide makes a real difference in mother, infant or family outcomes?

How do you know whether you and the people you work with are doing the right things? For example, what do you do about routine continuous electronic fetal monitoring; water birth; length of hospital stay for a healthy newborn infant; episiotomy? If you have a feeling that the current care you provide may not be the best practice or based on the latest scientific evidence, what do you do?

The challenge: Questions and actions

What is your practice? What is done in your setting? What is done in other centres?

If you are not sure about a particular 'intervention', perhaps the place to start is to find out the local norms of practice and the frequency of occurrence of the intervention in question. Are there differences between practitioners, disciplines or local institutions? Does the frequency differ between settings in other parts of the country or other countries? Major variation in the use of an intervention is often an indicator that the practice may not be justified. Keep in mind, however, that variation in practice may sometimes be legitimate and reflect differences between client populations.

If you know that data about the use of the intervention are regularly collected but not reported, for whatever reasons, it may be necessary for you to ask the keepers of the data (e.g. the health records department or the local health department, etc.) to do a special analysis of their data for you. In other cases, you may have access to the data, such as interventions reported in the birthing room logbook or your personal files, and you simply have to do the tabulations yourself. If no data exist, it might be necessary to start collecting descriptive data locally. An additional item on the usual prenatal care record or record of birth could be added. The collection of descriptive data might be a relevant project for a midwifery student in training. Linking with a student may provide fresh insight, and a willing pair of hands to actually do the descriptive detective work.

Where do you look for the evidence?

Physically locating the evidence about the effectiveness of an intervention can be challenging. The age-old method of hand searching the midwifery, nursing and medical literature is always an option, but the limitation with this approach is the number of journals you can feasibly scan and the possibility of overlooking an important study. One way around this is to conduct a computerized search of *MEDLINE*, the US National Library of Medicine's database, or *EMBase*, the European equivalent, to locate the literature on an intervention. This approach has the advantage of quickly accessing literally thousands of journals from around the world. As the number of databases available in libraries and strategies for searching are increasing, it is valuable to have an experienced librarian to assist with the selection of 'key words', sources and search strategies.

In addition, there are a number of places to turn to for assistance in finding midwifery literature. For example, there is MIDIRS, the Midwives Information and Resources Service, located in Bristol. The mission of MIDIRS is 'to be the central source of information relating to childbirth and to disseminate this information to midwives and others both nationally and internationally thereby contributing to the improvement of maternity care'. One of the activities of the organization is the MIDIRS Enquiry Service which provides literature searches of their database of over 42 000 references. MIDIRS has over 300 reading lists which contain the title of the relevant article, the author, where and when it was published and the original abstract. If the subject you are interested in is not listed, MIDIRS will, for a small fee, conduct a special tailor-made search to your requirements. MIDIRS also publishes quarterly the *MIDIRS Midwifery Digest* which selects information from over 550 journals. MIDIRS' services are available to midwives in the USA, Canada and Australia. For more information about how to contact MIDIRS and the costs of various services please refer to Appendix B.

Other compilations of the midwifery literature are the *Current Awareness Service (CAS)* distributed by the Royal College of Midwives, the *Royal College of Midwives' Midwifery Index*, and the *Index and Abstracts of the Current Literature* produced by the journal *Birth*.

There are also specialized midwifery research databases which should be consulted. One such database is the *Midwifery Research Database (MIRIAD)*. *MIRIAD* is a source book of midwifery research carried out in the UK, both completed and ongoing. The first edition of *MIRIAD* provided details on 267 studies (Simms *et al.*, 1994), with the second edition containing details of 99 new studies and updated information on 60 others (McCormick & Renfrew, 1996).

Once you have located the research about the intervention you are interested in, figuring out what the evidence means can be a challenge all its own. Depending on the topic and the skill of your searching, you may have discovered dozens of studies which may have used different methodologies and report different results. It is important to be able to differentiate good evidence, usually coming from systematic reviews, meta-analysis and RCTs, from poorer quality evidence, which is typically produced by non-experimental design studies such as non-randomized contemporaneous controls, formal comparisons with historic controls, case series and anecdotal reports. For practitioners with limited training in research methodology, evaluating the quality of the evidence of individual studies may be overwhelming. Keep in mind, however, that even experienced researchers sometimes debate vigorously about the quality of the evidence. If you have the interest and the time, you can learn the basics of research methods. Your local university or college library will have textbooks on conducting and evaluating research (e.g. Woods & Catanzaro, 1988; Polit & Hungler, 1995; Murphy-Black, 1993; Davies & Logan, 1994). A series published in the *Journal of the American Medical Association* entitled, 'User's guides to the medical literature' by the Evidence-Based Medicine Working Group is another source of information about how to read and interpret research reports (e.g. Oxman *et al.*, 1993; 1994; Guyatt *et al.*, 1994;

1995; Jaeschke *et al.*, 1994a; 1994b; Laupacis *et al.*, 1994; Hayward *et al.*, 1995; Richardson, *et al.*, 1995a; 1995b; Naylor *et al.*, 1996; in press; Wilson *et al.*, 1995).

Evaluating research needs to occur on a regular basis and is often better when done in a group, so you might also consider joining or forming a journal club. Journal clubs have a long history in medicine and usually involve small groups of practitioners and/or students meeting on an ongoing basis to discuss the latest literature. You might also consider approaching colleagues at the university as they may be willing to counsel you on how to assess the literature.

Fortunately there are at least two sources to which you can turn which may have already located the best available evidence about the intervention and systematically reviewed and synthesized it for you. One is *A Guide to Effective Care in Pregnancy and Childbirth (GECPC)* (Enkin *et al.*, 1995) and the other is the *Cochrane Library* (produced by the Cochrane Collaboration, Oxford). These two sources are by far the most important accumulation of scientific evidence about interventions in childbirth to date. As it almost always takes more than the results of one study to bring about change in practice, being able to make sense of the accumulation of research is essential.

GECPC provides the main conclusions of 40 systematic reviews of more than 500 published and unpublished RCTs of childbirth interventions which were reported in the *Cochrane Collaboration: Pregnancy and Childbirth Database (CCPCD)*, and first appeared in print form as *Effective Care in Pregnancy and Childbirth* (Chalmers *et al.*, 1989). The second edition of *GECPC* (Enkin *et al.*, 1995) is published by Oxford University Press and sells for around £12 (US $23). For practitioners interested in evidence-based practice and challenging obstetric interventions, the last chapter of *GECPC* which lists interventions (forms of care) by the availability of evidence is an excellent starting point (Enkin *et al.*, 1995). The chapter is divided into six types of interventions based on the evidence of effectiveness from controlled trials:

(1)   those that are beneficial;
(2)   those likely to be beneficial;
(3)   those with a trade-off between beneficial and adverse effects;
(4)   interventions of unknown effectiveness;
(5)   those unlikely to be beneficial; and
(6)   those likely to be ineffective or harmful.

The *Cochrane Library* took over from *CCPCD* in the summer of 1996 and includes quarterly updated systematic reviews of RCTs on CD-ROM. At present the *Cochrane Library* contains 63 reviews on interventions in pregnancy and childbirth. It also contains the citations to controlled trials on the pregnancy and childbirth specialized register plus citations contributed by other groups and those appearing in *MEDLINE*. Another useful component of the *Cochrane Library* is the *Cochrane Review of Methodology Database (CRMD)* which consists of a bibliography of articles on the science of research synthesis and on practical aspects of preparing systematic reviews. The *Cochrane Library* is relatively affordable at around £120 per year for a personal copy (US $200) and can be purchased from the *British Medical Journal* and other affiliated publishing centres including the American College of Physicians and the Canadian Medical Association.

Another source of current evidence about issues such as support in labour, fetal heart rate monitoring in labour, ultrasound screening, alcohol and pregnancy, and positions in labour and delivery is the series of *Informed Choice* leaflets produced by MIDIRS and the University of York National Health Service Centre for Reviews and Dissemination. These colourful and user-friendly leaflets summarize for women and professionals the most reliable evidence available and have been extensively peer reviewed by international experts. Another advantage of these documents is that they are the product of a multi-disciplinary effort and are supported by the Royal College of Midwives, the Royal College of General Practitioners and the Royal College of Obstetricians and Gynaecologists. The *Informed Choice* leaflets for women and the companion documents for professionals can be obtained from MIDIRS at a nominal fee of 30 pence per copy (US $0.50) plus postage. The development of leaflets on other topics are planned for the future.

When looking for a synthesis of the evidence about an intervention, you should also consider review articles. An example of good evidence-based review articles are those by Smith *et al.* (1991; 1993) on the management of normal delivery. Review articles can easily be retrieved in *MEDLINE* as they are indexed by the term 'review'. While the quality and thoroughness of review articles are variable, they are a good place to start to find related research and one author's interpretation of the evidence for practice.

Evidence-based practice guidelines developed by professional associations such as the Royal College of Obstetricians and Gynaecologists, the American College of Obstetricians and Gynecologists, the American College of Nurse-Midwives, the Society of Obstetricians and Gynecologists (Canada), the Obstetrical Interest Group of the North American Primary Care Research Group, and international bodies such as the World Health Organization may also provide a review of the scientific evidence about a particular intervention. These guidelines or consensus statements are usually produced by experts who have reviewed the evidence and come to a consensus. The consensus process frequently involves several drafts and input from many people and vigorous debate. Therefore practice guidelines can be a particularly valuable resource.

Consumer groups are yet another source to consider when looking for evidence about a particular intervention. Groups such as the AIMS, the NCT and the ICEA often collect the evidence on interventions and sometimes even publish reviews along with position statements. For example, the ICEA has position papers on the use of diagnostic ultrasound during pregnancy, epidural anaesthesia for labour, Caesarean birth, and vaginal birth after Caesarean birth (VBAC).

What is the scientific evidence for the intervention?

Once you have located, or tried to locate, the evidence about the intervention, the next step is making a decision about what the evidence says and whether it applies in your setting. Generally speaking, the evidence will fall into one of three broad categories: it simply doesn't exist, the evidence is mixed or weak, or there is strong evidence about the intervention.

Little or no evidence

If despite all your looking you find little or no scientific evidence about the intervention, you have at least two options. You can gather your own evidence by conducting research yourself or you can encourage others to do research by raising the question with researchers.

As has been seen with the case of episiotomy, one strategy for encouraging researchers to undertake research is to ask questions that highlight the lack of evidence about the intervention. For a widely accepted or routine intervention, the key is to raise doubts in practitioners' and researchers' minds about the rationale for the intervention, which may have come to be taken-for-granted in your setting or within midwifery more generally. Focus attention on the intervention by revealing the lack of evidence for the intervention and asking questions about why this intervention is being performed. Increasing awareness of the intervention encourages practitioners to think about their use of the intervention and may provoke researchers to study the issue.

Writing letters to the editor of professional journals is one way of reaching many practitioners and researchers at the same time. Another approach might be to try to convince a journal editor to devote an editorial to highlighting the need for research about the intervention. Writing letters to funding agencies, government health agencies and hospital authorities describing the lack of research and asking what they intend to do about the paucity of research on the intervention is another strategy.

Involving the media, childbirth activists and organizations, as well as childbearing women in questioning the intervention and lack of research for it may also be a very effective means of helping to create an environment supportive of researchers studying the intervention. For example, childbirth organizations can often challenge and ask questions without penalty. This approach gives some health professionals the opportunity of supporting consumers and their questioning while at the same avoiding the perception that they are challenging the practices of their own profession.

Asking questions, involving others in the questioning and generally raising awareness of the issues are all strategies that can also be useful in influencing funders to make research of the intervention a priority. Unless researchers have their studies funded, they cannot undertake research.

Mixed or weak evidence

After systematically reviewing the literature, it is very common to find inconclusive evidence for an intervention. This is more likely to occur when the studies that have been undertaken are small and use non-experimental (observational) designs. However, even the results from RCTs sometimes greatly differ, making it difficult to come to a conclusion about the effectiveness of an intervention. When the evidence for an intervention is mixed, what is needed is more research. In some settings, it may be sufficient to gather local evidence by conducting your own study or pilot study. In other cases, encouraging researchers to conduct more and better studies on the intervention is the way to go. The same strategies suggested for when there is no evidence available can be adopted when the evidence is mixed. Here, however, increasing awareness and creating controversy may be somewhat easier because of the published lack of certainty about what is best.

In the meantime, however, decisions still have to be made about whether or not to use the intervention. In light of the ambiguity of the evidence, the best approach is to inform women of the existing evidence and support their informed choice.

Strong evidence that the intervention is beneficial or harmful

Change your own practice
Once you have determined there is convincing evidence of the effectiveness of an intervention, the first step is to bring your own practice into line with the research findings. While ultimately you make the decision about what you do, changing the way you practise may not be

as simple as it sounds. On a psychological level, fear of the unknown or fear of failure may discourage you from changing. Not doing something you have been taught to do and have done for years or trying something for the first time may require considerable courage and a high tolerance of ambiguity. Neither of these characteristics come easily to most people.

Strategies for overcoming psychological barriers to change include talking to others who have successfully used the intervention, developing new skills by going to another centre for training, watching a demonstration video, or observing a role model. With the example of episiotomy, seeking out other midwives who perform very few episiotomies and asking how they achieve this and what problems they encounter may be sufficient to encourage some to try avoiding episiotomy more often. Another strategy is to try out the intervention for a short period of time before you commit yourself to changing. This affords you an opportunity to gain experience with the proposed intervention. Once again, offering women the choice is essential. You may find that getting your client's perspective about their experience with the intervention can direct and reinforce change.

Attempt to change colleagues' practices in your setting
As the case study of episiotomy has shown, there are also practical issues such as the prevalent belief system, the availability of technology and resources, institutional policies and local norms of practice, peer pressure, professional and intra-professional concerns, and legal concerns which can also serve as major impediments to your adopting or abandoning an intervention. You are part of a social system and this means you may be subjected to considerable influences. Identify these influences and attempt to address them where this is possible and feasible.

How can you bring about change in your setting? You first have to publicize the evidence about the intervention which means telling your colleagues about the research. If they are unaware of the research findings, they cannot be expected to change. Tell co-workers about the research, give them copies of the journal article, arrange for the researchers to come and give a talk about their results, put the paper on the reading list of the journal club. Think of innovative ways to get the research into the hands of your co-workers and clients and actively involve them in the process of bringing about change. For the change process to be successful it is important to actively involve those thinking about adopting the proposed innovation.

As was seen with some of the more recent research focusing on lowering the use of episiotomy (Henriksen *et al.*, 1994; Reynolds, 1995), introducing the intervention into the Continuous Quality Improvement (CQI) or Continuous Quality Assurance (CQA) programme may be a useful method of bringing about and maintaining change. The CQI/CQA programme in your institution may be of benefit to help you monitor the intervention in question and the related outcomes. These programmes often involve multi-disciplinary peer review with chart audits and a regular reporting system.

Next, you need to identify the barriers to the proposed change and work to minimize them. At the same time, identify the factors that you can use to facilitate change, such as people who are positive toward the intervention, the beneficial outcomes that might be achieved, or the impact on resources. You may be surprised what support exists for the intervention when you start looking for it. Anticipate problems. For example, if the existing belief system is at odds with the proposed changed, it may be necessary to simultaneously modify the belief system to make it more congruent with the proposed change. If a hospital policy is a barrier to the adoption of the proposed change you may need to work on changing the policy. If the proposed change simplifies work in some way, promote this characteristic of the change. If the proposed change has the potential for cost savings make this known as managers are always looking for ways to economize.

To bring about change successfully, you need to identify potential agents of change and make use of them. These individuals may be highly respected colleagues, other professionals, clients, the media, local ministry of health officials, or managers. Decision makers such as managers for example can be extremely effective agents of change, so try to see how the proposed change might be viewed through their eyes. Remember that managers may be interested in the proposed change for reasons in addition to the results of research showing that the intervention is effective. While this in itself may not necessarily be a bad thing, these other factors do impact on their enthusiasm for the proposed change and so it may be necessary to anticipate these factors and address them early on.

Again, the strategy of piloting or trying out the proposed change for a limited period of time may be an effective means of sensitizing colleagues to the intervention and offering them the opportunity to gain experience with it before committing themselves to adopting it permanently. Having group discussions about the pros and cons of the proposed change and experiences with it may also be useful in developing new norms around the practice.

Attempt to change the profession
While most of your energy may be directed toward bringing about change in your local environment, there is also the profession as a whole which might also benefit from being challenged. Clearly, challenging the profession requires ambitious, far-reaching efforts, but as

the case of episiotomy has shown, individual practitioners and researchers can make a difference.

Writing editorials and letters to the editors of journals can be an effective way of initially creating uncertainty about the effectiveness of interventions or highlighting the strength of evidence for an intervention. Publishing research about interventions and undertaking implementation studies of interventions are critical for advancing evidence-based practice. Working to get practice guidelines developed for the intervention is another method of bringing the profession's attention to the proposed change, as is participating in task forces. Other strategies for bringing about change in the profession include introducing the proposed change into the midwifery school curricula and midwifery textbooks once there is sufficient evidence for the intervention.

Be persistent

If your initial efforts to bring about change are to no avail, you have two choices: you can live with things the way they are or you can keep working to bring about change. If you choose the latter, continue lobbying, remember that you only need a critical mass of like-minded practitioners to make a difference. Move slowly. Incremental change is often easier to introduce than sudden radical change. Also, pick your battles carefully.

To challenge or not to challenge?

While rewards are usually substantial, challenging obstetric interventions may not always be easy and sometimes requires fortitude and patience. It can lead to considerable stress and interpersonal distress dealing with colleagues. For example, several of the key informants interviewed for this book described the 'abuse' they suffered from colleagues who strongly believed in the practice they were challenging. As one of them noted, there were times when she felt 'really despised and rejected and totally lonely'. While the key informants understood why others responded this way to their challenging, 'I appreciate I can be very threatening because I'm shaking the ground under their feet', it did not make it any less hurtful for them.

Now perhaps you are beginning to think, 'Why bother? After all I am just one person and what difference would it make if I questioned "tradition" in my setting?' Fortunately for science, there are still plenty of professionals and consumers who question current practices and challenge the health care system. However, do not forget that the real reason for doing this is to improve the health of mothers, infants, families and society and to ensure the profession provides the care known to be the most effective. As one of the key informants noted:

> '... it doesn't take much to keep me going, it just takes the odd letter from a woman, it doesn't happen very often but it is enough to say "thank you". And I think, well that's why I'm doing it really. Because you are not doing it for the managers or the obstetricians, you are doing it for the woman at the receiving end and her baby.'

For many of the key informants, talking with women and hearing what they are saying keeps them on track and gives them strength to continue challenging obstetric interventions. While challenging obstetric interventions may be difficult and appear at times thankless, the quest for the best care possible can also be energizing, with professional and personal rewards.

Appendix A

Statistics

The Prevalence of Episiotomy in England, Wales and the USA (1967–1993)

(See also Fig. 3.)

Number of episiotomies per 100 vaginal deliveries

Year		England and Wales		USA
		Primips	Multips	
1967	25.0			*
68	*			*
69	*			*
1970	*			*
71	*			*
72	*			*
73	44.0			*
74	47.4			*
75	48.6			*
76	50.6			*
77	52.0			*
78	53.4			*
79	*			65.1
1980	52.2	70.5	38.3	64.0
81	*			64.0
82	*			63.1
83	*			61.2
84	43[2]			61.1
85	36.6[1]	54.6[1]	22.8[1]	61.1
86	*			60.8
87	*			61.9
88	*			59.0
89	36[2]			56.8
1990	*			55.8
91	*			55.4
92	*			53.9
93	*			50.4

* Not available

[1] Data for England only
[2] Survey data, not population data (Fleissig, 1993)

Sources: Macfarlane & Mugford, 1984; Department of Health and Social Security, and Office of Population Censuses and Surveys Welsh Office, 1986; Department of Health, and Office of Population Censuses and Surveys, 1988; Kozak, 1989; Fleissig, 1993; National Center for Health Statistics, 1992–1995.

Changes in Obstetrical Practices in England and Wales, 1967–78 (see also Fig. 4)

Year	Hospital Deliveries (%)[1]	Episiotomy (%)[2]	Induced (%)[1]	Instruments (forceps) (%)[1]
1967	80.6	25	16.8	7.5
1968	–	–	18	7.9
1969	–	–	20.3	8.2
1970	–	–	23.2	8.8
1971	–	–	26.3	9.4
1972	–	–	29.2	10.5
1973	–	44	34.9	11
1974	–	47.4	38.9	12
1975	94.9	48.6	35	12.1
1976	95.9	50.6	35.5	13
1977	96.5	52	36.8	13.4
1978	97.1	53.4	36.3	13.3

[1] % of all births
[2] % of vaginal births

Source: Macfarlane & Mugford, 1984.

Episiotomy Rate, Oxford Radcliffe NHS Trust Hospital, 1980–84 (see also Fig. 5)

	Primips (%)[1]	Multips (%)[1]
1980	72.6	36.8
1981	69.9	33.9
1982	58.7	24.9
1983	49.8	21.3
1984	44.9	15.4

[1] % of vaginal births

Source: Reynolds & Yudkin, 1987.

Appendix B

Useful Addresses

AIMS
Beverley Lawrence Beech
Honorary Chair
21 Iver Lane
Iver
Buckinghamshire SL0 91H
Tel: 01753-652781
Fax: 01753-654142

American College of Nurse-Midwives
818 Connecticut Avenue NW
Suite 900
Washington DC
USA 20006
Tel.: 202-728-9860
Fax: 202-728-9897

The American College of Nurse-Midwives produces *FACTS* sheets which discuss the research evidence for numerous maternity care practices.

American College of Obstetricians and Gynecologists
409 12th Street SW
Washington DC
USA 20024-2188

The American College of Obstetricians and Gynecologists in collaboration with the American Academy of Pediatrics produce *Guidelines for Perinatal Care.*

Current Awareness Service (CAS)
The Librarian
Royal College of Midwives
15 Mansfield Street
London W1M 0BE

ICEA
PO Box 20048
Minneapolis
Minnesota
USA 55420-0048
Tel: 612-854-8660
Fax: 612-854-8772
E-mail: info@icea.org
Internet: http://www.icea.org

MIRIAD – Midwifery Research Database
Midwifery Studies
University of Leeds
22 Hyde Terrace
Leeds LS2 9LN
Tel.: 0113-233-6886
Fax: 0113-244-9730
E-mail: feliciam@epid.leeds.ac.uk

MIDIRS – Midwives Information and Resources Service
9 Elmdale Road
Bristol BS8 1SL
Tel.: 0117-925-1791
Fax: 0117-925-1792
Freephone in UK: 0800-581009
E-mail: midirs@dial.pipex.com
Internet: http://www.gn.apc.org/midirs

MIDIRS Midwifery Digest
Subscription rates:

UK:

Personal subscriber	£34
Institutions	£60

Worldwide:

Personal subscriber	£42
Institutions	£65

MIDIRS Enquiry Service
Personal subscribers to *MIDIRS Midwifery Digest*:

	Reading List	Special Search
Personal subscriber	£3.95	£5.50
Institutions	£4.95	£6.50
All others:		
UK	£10.00	£15.00
Worldwide	£11.00	£16.00

Informed Choice leaflets can be purchased from MIDIRS.

NCT
Alexandra House
Oldham Terrace
Acton
London W3 6NH
Tel: 0181-992-6837
Fax: 0181-992-5929

World Health Organization
Headquarters
1211 Geneva 27
Switzerland
Tel.: 22-791-2111
Fax: 22-791-0746
E-mail: inf@who.ch
Internet: http://www.who.ch

Regional Office for Europe
Scherfigovej 8
DK 2100
Copenhagen
Denmark
Tel.: 39-17-17-17
Fax: 39-17-18-18

Regional Office for the Americas
Pan American Sanitary Bureau
525 23rd Street NW
Washington DC
USA 20037
Tel.: 202-861-3200
Fax: 202-223-5971
Internet: http://www.paho.org

References

AAOG (1920) List of Fellows. *Transactions of the American Association of Obstetricians and Gynecologists*, XXI–XLVIII.

AAOG (1942) List of Fellows. *Transactions of the American Association of Obstetricians, Gynecologists and Abdominal Surgeons*, **LIV**: IX–LI.

Adamson, L. (1978) Unkind Cuts. *The Guardian*, 1 November, 9.

AGS (1885) List of Fellows. *Transactions of the American Gynecological Society*, **10**, 12–19.

AGS (1904) List of Fellows. *Transactions of the American Gynecological Society*, **29**, XVI–XXVII.

AGS (1915) List of Fellows. *Transactions of the American Gynecological Society*, **40**, XVI–XXIX.

AGS (1952) List of Fellows. *Transactions of the American Gynecological Society*, **74**, IX–XLII.

AGS (1982) List of Fellows. *Transactions of the American Gynecological Society*, **104**, X–XXXI.

Ahn, M. O., Cha, K. Y. & Phelan, J. (1992) The low birth weight infant: is there a preferred route of delivery? *Clinics in Perinatology*, **19** (June), 411–23.

AIMS Quarterly Newsletter (1976) Report of a meeting between representatives of AIMS and Maternity Services Department of the DHSS, 5 March. June, 6–10.

Alden, L. (1979) *Postpartum evaluation of delivery with or without episiotomy*. Master's thesis, University of Illinois at the Medical Center, Chicago.

Aldridge, A. & Watson, P. (1935) Analysis of end-results of labor in primiparas after spontaneous versus prophylactic methods of delivery. *American Journal of Obstetrics and Gynecology*, **30**, 554–65.

Anderson, S. (1977) Childbirth as a pathological process: an American perspective. *American Journal of Maternal and Child Nursing*, July/August, 240–4.

Anderson, R. & Greener, D. (1991) A descriptive analysis of home births attended by CNMs in two nurse-midwifery services. *Journal of Nurse-Midwifery*, **36**(2), 95–103.

Anisef, P. & Basson, P. (1979) The institutionalization of a profession. *Sociology of Work and Occupations*, **6**(3), 353–72.

Anonymous (1968) Episiotomy. Editorial. *Lancet*, 13 January, 75–6.

Anonymous (1973) Pain after birth. Editorial. *British Medical Journal*, 8 December, 565.

Anonymous (1974) A time to be born. Editorial. *Lancet*, 16 November, 1183–4.

Anonymous (1976) Episiotomy – the unkindest cut. *AIMS Quarterly Newsletter*, March, 7.

Anonymous (1979) Unkind Cuts. *AIMS Quarterly Newsletter*, Summer, 7.

Anonymous (1985) Episiotomy and third-degree tears. Editorial. *Lancet*, 5 October, 760.

Anonymous (1993a) Mothers who use nurse midwives have fewer C-sections, episiotomies and shorter hospital stays. *Journal of Nursing Administration*, **23** (7/8), 11–12.

Anonymous (1993b) Mothers who use nurse midwives have fewer C-sections, episiotomies and shorter hospital stays. *Pennsylvania Nurse*, **48** (4), 9.

Anspach, B. (1915a) The value of a more frequent employment of episiotomy in the second stage. Paper read before the American Gynecological Society. *American Journal of Obstetrics and Diseases of Women and Children*, **72**, 711–14.

Anspach (1915b) The value of a more frequent employment of episiotomy in the second stage of labor. *Transactions of the American Gynecological Society*, **40**, 14–18.

Anspach (1923) The trend of modern obstetrics: what is the danger? How can it be changed? *Transactions of the American Gynecological Society*, **48**, 96–105, Discussion 105–108.

Anthony, S., Buitendijk, S. E., Zondervan, K. T., van Rijssel, E. J. & Verkerk, P. H. (1994) Episiotomies and the occurrence of severe perineal lacerations. *British Journal of Obstetrics and Gynaecology*, **101** (12), 1065–7.

Applegate, J. C. (1924) Rational obstetrics from the teaching viewpoint. *Journal of Obstetrics and Gynecology*, **7**, 181–8, Discussion 222–5.

Argentine Episiotomy Trial Collaborative Group (1993) Routine vs selective episiotomy: a randomised controlled trial. *Lancet*, **342**, 1517–18.

Arms, S. (1975a) *Immaculate Deception*. Houghton Mifflin, New York.

Arms, S. (1975b) How hospitals complicate childbirth. *Ms*, **8** (May), 108–15.

Arms, S. (1981) *Immaculate Deception*, 3rd edn. Bantam Books, New York.

Arney, W. R. (1985) *Power and the Profession of Obstetrics*. University of Chicago Press, Chicago.

Arthure, H. G. E. (1970) Repair of the perineum. Letter to the Editor. *Lancet*, 27 June, 1405.

Avery, M. & Burket, B. (1986) Effect of perineal massage on the incidence of episiotomy and perineal laceration in a nurse-midwifery service. *Journal of Nurse-Midwifery*, **31** (May/June), 128–34.

Avery, M. & Van Arsdale, L. (1987) Perineal massage. Effect on the incidence of episiotomy and laceration in a nulliparous population. *Journal of Nurse-Midwifery*, **32** (May/June), 181–4.

Balaskas, J. (1989) *New Active Birth. A Concise Guide to Natural Childbirth*. Unwin, London.

Ballentyne, J. W. (1919) The protection of the perineum in labour. Critical review. *Edinburgh Medical Journal*, **23**, 407–13.

Ballew, J. & Sullivan, R. (1958) Third degree lacerations in obstetrics: cause and effect. *General Practitioner*, **17** (2), 102–105.

Banister, J.B. et al. (1927) *The Queen Charlotte's Practice of Obstetrics*. J.&A. Churchill, London.

Banta, H. D. (1983) Social science research on medical technology: utility and limitations. *Social Science and Medicine*, **17** (18), 1363–9.

Banta, H. D. (1984) Embracing or rejecting innovations: clinical diffusion of health care technology. In: *The Machine at the Bedside* (ed. S. J. Reiser), pp. 65–85. Cambridge University Press, New York.

Banta, H. D. (1989) National strategies for promoting effective care. In: *Effective Care in Pregnancy and Childbirth* (eds I. Chalmers, M. Enkin & M. Keirse), pp. 1453–6. Oxford University Press, Oxford.

Banta, H. D., Behney, C. J. & Sisk Willems, J. (1981) *Toward Rational Technology in Medicine. Considerations for Health Policy*. Springer, New York.

Banta, H. D. & Thacker, S. B. (1979) Policies toward medical technology: the case of electronic fetal monitoring. *American Journal of Public Health*, **69** (September), 931–5.

Banta, H. D. & Thacker, S. B. (1982) The risk and benefits of episiotomy: a review. Paper presented at the Second Conference on Technological Approaches to Obstetrics: Benefits, Risks, Alternatives, San Francisco, California, 16 October 1981. *Birth. Issues in Perinatal Care and Education*, **9** (spring), 25–30.

Banta, H. D. & Thacker, S. B. (1990) The case for reassessment of health care technology. Once is not enough. *Journal of the American Medical Association*, **264** (11 July), 235–40.

Barker, F. (1874) *The Puerperal Diseases. Clinical Lectures Delivered at Bellevue Hospital*. D. Appleton, New York.

Barker, (1981) The unkindest cut of all. Disputation. *World Medicine*, 8 August, 40–41.

Barter, R., Parks, J. & Tyndal, C. (1960) Median episiotomies and complete lacerations. Address of the Guest Speaker, presented at the Annual Meeting of the South Atlantic Association of Obstetricians and Gynecologists, Hollywood, Florida, 31 January to 3 February. *American Journal of Obstetrics and Gynecology*, **80** (October), 654–62.

Baruffi, G., Dellinger, W., Gibson Timmons, R. & Ross, A. (1984) Patterns of obstetric procedures' use in maternity care. *Obstetrics and Gynecology,* **64** (October), 493–8.

Beacham, W. Davis (1953) The American Academy of Obstetrics and Gynecology: First Presidential Address. A history of American obstetric and gynecologic organizations and the genesis of the American Academy. *Obstetrics and Gynecology,* **1** (January), 115–24.

Bean, C. (1972) *Methods of Childbirth: A Complete Guide to Childbirth Classes and Maternity Care.* Doubleday and Co., Garden City, New York.

Bean, C. (1982) *Methods of Childbirth,* revised edn. Dolphin Books, Garden City, New York.

Beazley, J. M. (1986) Maternal injuries and complications. In: *Dewhurst's Textbook of Obstetrics and Gynaecology for Postgraduates* (ed. C. R. Whitfield), pp. 417. Blackwell Scientific Publications, Oxford.

Beech, B. Lawrence (1987a) Birth is not an illness. *AIMS Quarterly Journal,* Spring, 1–2.

Beech, B. Lawrence (1987b) *Who's Having Your Baby? A Health Rights Handbook for Maternity Care.* Camden Press, London.

Beech, B. Lawrence (1991) *Who's Having Your Baby? A Health Rights Handbook for Maternity Care,* 2nd edn., Bedford Square Press, London.

Beech, B. Lawrence (ed) (1996) *Water Birth Unplugged – Proceedings of the First International Water Birth Conference.* Books for Midwives Press, Hale, Cheshire.

Bell, S. E. (1986) A new model of medical technology development: a case study of DES. In: *The Adoption and Social Consequences of Medical Technologies* (eds J. Roth & S. Burt Ruzek), pp. 1–32. *Research in Sociology of Health Care – A Research Annual,* Vol. 4. JAI Press, Greenwich, Connecticut.

Bell, S. E. (1989) Technology in medicine: development, diffusion, and health policy. In: *Handbook of Medical Sociology* (eds H. Freeman & L. Sol), pp. 185–204. Prentice Hall, Englewood Cliffs, New Jersey.

Bennett, V. R. & Brown, L. K. (eds) (1989) *Myles Textbook for Midwives,* 11th edn. Churchill Livingstone, Edinburgh.

Berlind, M. M. (1932) Episiotomy in prematurity as a prevention against cerebral hemorrhage. *Medical Journal and Record,* **135** (17 February), 180–82.

Beynon, L. (1973) Some surgical procedures in obstetrics. *Nursing Mirror and Midwives Journal,* **136** (13 April), 23–6.

Beynon, C. L. (1982) Episiotomy. Letter to the Editor. *British Medical Journal,* **284** (20 February), 594–5.

Bill, A. (1932) The newer obstetrics. Presidential Address to the American Association of Obstetricians, Gynecologists and Abdominal Surgeons, White Sulphur Springs, Virginia, 14–16 September 1931. *Journal of Obstetrics and Gynecology,* **23**(2), 155–64.

Blevins, W. J. (1929) Episiotomy with Modified Operative Technic. Paper read before the meeting of the California Northern District Medical Society, 10 April 1928. *American Journal of Obstetrics and Gynecology,* **17,** 197–204.

Blondel, B. & Kaminski, M. (1985) Episiotomy and third-degree tears. Letter to the Editor. *British Journal of Obstetrics and Gynaecology,* **92,** 1297–8.

Borgatta, L., Piening, P. & Cohen, W. (1989) Association of episiotomy and delivery position with deep perineal laceration during spontaneous delivery in nulliparaous women. *American Journal of Obstetrics and Gynecology,* **160** (February), 194–297.

Boston Women's Health Book Collective (1973) *Our Bodies, Ourselves. A Book by and for Women.* Simon and Schuster, New York.

Boston Women's Health Book Collective (1976) *Our Bodies, Ourselves. A Book by and for Women,* 2nd edn completely revised and expanded. Simon and Schuster, New York.

Boston Women's Health Book Collective (1984) *The New Our Bodies, Ourselves.* Simon and Schuster, New York.

Bowe, N. (1981) Intact perineum: a slow delivery of the head does not adversely affect the outcome of the newborn. *Journal of Nurse-Midwifery,* **26** (March/April), 5–11.

Boyd, C. & Sellers, L. (1982) *The British Way of Birth.* Introduction by Esther Rantzen. Pan Books, London.

Brackbill, Y., Rice, J. & Young, D. (1984) *Birth Trap*. Warner Books, St Louis.

Bradley, R. (1981). *Husband-coached Childbirth*, 3rd edn. Foreword by Ashley Montagu. Harper and Row, New York.

Brendsel, C., Peterson, G. & Mehl, L. (1979) Episiotomy: facts, fictions, figures, and alternatives. In: *Compulsory Hospitalization. Freedom of Choice in Childbirth? Vol. 1* (eds D. Stewart & L. Stewart), pp. 169–75. NAPSAC, Marble Hill, Missouri.

Brendsel, C., Peterson, G. & Mehl, L. (1980) Routine episiotomy and pelvic symptomatology. *Women and Health*, **5** (Winter), 59–60.

Brendsel, C., Peterson, G. & Mehl, L. (1981) The role of episiotomy in pelvic symptomatology. In: *Episiotomy: Physical and Emotional Aspects* (ed. S. Kitzinger), pp. 36–44. National Childbirth Trust, London.

Bright Banister, J., Bourne, A., Davies, T. *et al.* (1927) *Queen Charlotte's Text-Book of Obstetrics*. J. and A. Churchill, London.

Bright Banister, J., Bourne, A., Davies, T. *et al.* (1956) *Queen Charlotte's Text-Book of Obstetrics*, 9th edn. J. and A. Churchill, London.

British Medical Association (1936) The BMA and maternity services. *British Medical Journal*, **1**, 656.

Brody, H. & Thompson, J. (1981) The Maximin strategy in modern obstetrics. *Journal of Family Practice*, **12**(6), 977–86.

Bromberg, M. (1986) Presumptive maternal benefits of routine episiotomy. A literature review. *Journal of Nurse-Midwifery*, **31** (May/June), 121–7.

Bromwich, P. D. (1981) Episiotomy. Letter to the Editor. *Midwife, Health Visitor and Community Nurse*, **17** (April).

Broomall, A. (1878) The operation of episiotomy as a prevention of perineal ruptures during labor. Paper read before the Obstetrical Society of Philadelphia by A. H. Smith, 7 February 1878. *American Journal of Obstetrics and Diseases of Women and Children*, **11**, 517–25, 605–607.

Broun, L. (ed.) (1918) *Album of the Fellows of the American Gynecological Society 1876–1917*. Wm. J. Dornan, Printer, Philadelphia.

Buchan, P. & Nicholls, J. (1980) Pain after episiotomy – a comparison of two methods of repair. *Journal of the Royal College of General Practitioners*, **30** (May), 297–300.

Bucher, R. (1988) On the natural history of health care occupations. *Work and Occupations*, **15**(2), 131–47.

Buekens, P., Lagasse, R. & Wollast, E. (1986) Episiotomy and third-degree tears. Letter to the Editor. *Lancet*, 22 February, **1**, 441.

Buekens, P., Lagasse, R., Dramaix, M. & Wollast, E. (1985) Episiotomy and third-degree tears. *British Journal of Obstetrics and Gynaecology*, **92**, 820–23.

Burkhardt, P. (1978) Letter to the Editor. *Journal of Nurse-Midwifery*, **23** (Spring/Summer), 22–3.

Buxbaum, H. (1936) Out-patient obstetrics. A review of 6 863 cases. Paper read before the Chicago Gynecological Society, 17 May 1935. *American Journal of Obstetrics and Gynecology*, **31**, 409–19.

Byford, H. T. (1920) Discussion of DeLee's paper entitled, 'The Prophylactic Forceps Operation'. *American Journal of Obstetrics and Gynecology*, **1** (1), 78.

Cameron, J. Chalmers (1903) Instrumental operations. In: *The Text-book of Obstetrics* (eds R. Norris & R. Dickinson), pp. 392–460. W. B. Saunders and Co., Philadelphia.

Campbell, R. & Macfarlane, A. (1987) *Where to Be Born? The Debate and the Evidence*. p. 14 National Perinatal Epidemiology Unit, Oxford.

Carter, L. (1984) A little knowledge. Midwifery Forum. *Nursing Mirror*, **159** (26 September), i–ix.

Chadwick, J. (1881) Obstetric and gynaecology literature, 1876–1881. Address in Obstetrics and Diseases of Women at the Annual Meeting of the American Medical Association 3–6 May 1881. *Transactions of the American Medical Association*, **32**, 253–65.

Chadwick, J., Dickinson, R. & Edgar, J. Clifton (eds) (1901) *Album of the Fellows of the American Gynecological Society 1876–1900*. Wm. J. Dornan, Printer, Philadelphia.

Chalmers, B. (1995) Psychosomatic obstetrics in the countries of Central and Eastern Europe. *Journal of Psychosomatic Obstetrics and Gynecology*, **16**, 59–63.

Chalmers, I. (1975) Evaluation of different approaches to obstetric care. Paper presented at Warwick University, 10 October 1975.

Chalmers, I. (1976a) British debate on obstetric practice. *Pediatrics*, **58**(3), 308–12.

Chalmers, I. (1976b) Obstetric practice and outcome of pregnancy in Cardiff residents 1965–73. *British Medical Journal*, **1**, 735–8.

Chalmers, I., Enkin, M. & Keirse, M. (eds) (1989) *Effective Care in Pregnancy and Childbirth*. Oxford University Press, Oxford.

Chambliss, L., Daly, C., Medearis, A., Ames, M., Kayne, M. & Paul, R. (1992) The role of selection bias in comparing Cesarean birth rates between physician and midwifery management. *Obstetrics and Gynecology*, **80**(2), 161–5.

Chassar Moir, J. (1974) Pain after birth. Letter to the Editor. *British Medical Journal*, **901** (9 February), 242–3.

Child, C. G. Jr (1919) Episiotomy: its relation to the proper conduct of the perineal stage of labor. Paper read before the City (Charity) Hospital Alumni Society, 19 March 1919. *Medical Record*, **96** (26 July), 142–4.

Chimura, T. (1985) Routine use of episiotomy and its problems. *Josanpu Zasshi*, **39** (9), 790–93.

Cianfrani, T. (1960) *A Short History of Obstetrics and Gynecology*. Charles C. Thomas, Springfield, Massachusetts.

Cochrane, S. (1992) Perineal trauma. *Nursing Times*, **88** (20 May), 64.

Cockersell, S. M. (1982) Episiotomy. Letter to the Editor. *British Medical Journal*, **284** (6 February), 425.

Cogan, R. & Edmunds, E. (1977) The unkindest cut of all? *Contemporary OB/GYN*, **9** (April), 55–60.

Cogan, R. & Edmunds, E. (1978) The unkindest cut of all? *Journal of Nurse-Midwifery*, **23** (Spring/Summer), 17–21.

Cohen, L. & Rothschild, H. (1979) The bandwagons of medicine. *Perspectives in Biology and Medicine*, Spring, 531–8.

Colette, C. (1991), [Consequences of a deliberate fluctuation in the number of episiotomies.] *Revue Française de Gynecologie et D'Obstetrique*, **86**(4), 303–305.

Combs, C. A., Robertson, P. & Laros, R. (1990) Risk factors for third-degree and fourth-degree perineal lacerations in forceps and vacuum deliveries. *American Journal of Obstetrics and Gynecology*, **163** (1), 100–104.

Conn, L. C., Vant, J. R. & Cantor, M. (1941) A critical analysis of blood loss in 2000 obstetric cases. Paper read before the Annual Meeting of the American Gynecological Assocaition, Colorado Springs, 26–28 May 1941. *American Journal of Obstetrics and Gynecology*, **52**, 768–81, Discussion 781–5.

Cooke, W. R. (1937) Management of birth injuries. *American Journal of Surgery*, **35** (2), 409–16.

Coquatrix, N. (1985) [Episiotomy and Sexual Mutilations.] *Nursing Quebec*, **5** (March–April), 22–6.

Coquatrix, N. (1987) *Épisiotomie. Les Grands Sous-entends d'une Petite Coupure*. Les Presses de L'Université de Montréal, Montreal.

Cosner, K. R., Dougherty, M. & Bishop, K. (1991a) Dynamic characteristics of the circumvaginal muscles during pregnancy and the postpartum. *Journal of Nurse-Midwifery*, **36** (4), 221–5.

Cosner, K. R., Doughterty, M. & Bishop, K. (1991b) Pelvic muscles and episiotomy. *American Journal of Obstetrics and Gynecology*, **164** (3), 936.

Cottrell, B. & Davies Shannahan, M. (1986) Effect of the birth chair on duration of second stage labor and maternal outcome. *Nursing Research*, **35** (6), 364–7.

Crawford, J. S. (1982) Episiotomy. Letter to the Editor. *British Medical Journal*, **284** (20 February), 594.

Crawford, L., Quint, E. & Pearl, M. (1993) Incontinence following rupture of the anal sphincter during delivery. *Obstetrics and Gynecology*, **82** (October), 527–31.

Credé, C. & Colpe (1884) Ueb er die Zweckmässigkeit der einseitigen seitlichen Incision beim Dannschutzverfahren. *Archiv für Gynäkologie*, **24**, 148–68.

Cunningham, C. B. & Pilkington, J. W. (1955) Complete Perineotomy. Paper read before the Annual Meeting of the South Atlantic Association of Obstetricians and Gynecologists, Williamsburg, Virginia, 10–12 February 1955. *American Journal of Obstetrics and Gynecology*, **70** (6), 1225–31.

Cunningham, F. G., MacDonald, P. & Gant, N. (1989) *Williams Obstetrics*, 18th edn. Appleton & Lange, Norwalk, Connecticut.

Cunningham, F. G., MacDonald, P., Gant, N., Leveno, K. & Gilstrap, L. (1993) *Williams Obstetrics*, 19th edn. Appleton & Lange, Norwalk, Connecticut.

Dallas, D. A. (1953) The routine use of episiotomy with a description of the continuous knotless repair. *Western Journal of Surgery, Obstetrics and Gynecology*, **61** (January), 29–35.

Danforth, D. C. (1922) Is conservative obstetrics to be abandoned? *American Journal of Obstetrics and Gynecology*, **3**, 609–16.

Danforth, D. N. (1974) Contemporary Titans: Joseph Bolivar DeLee and Whitridge Williams. Presidential Address, American Gynecological Society, May 1974. *American Journal of Obstetrics and Gynecology*, **120** (November), 577–88.

Danforth, W. C. (1928) Immediate repair of the cervix after labor. *American Journal of Obstetrics and Gynecology*, **15**, 505–65.

Dannreuther, W. (1931) The American Board of Obstetrics and Gynecology. Its organization, function and objectives. *Journal of the American Medical Association*, **96** (10), 797–8.

David, M. (1993) Wer erfand den Dammschnitt? Zur Geschichte der Episiotomie [Who invented the episiotomy? On the history of episiotomy]. *Zentralblatt Für Gynakologie*, **115** (4), 188–93.

Davies, B. & Logan, J. (1994) *Reading Research. A User-friendly Guide for Nurses and Other Health Professionals*. Canadian Nurses Association, Ottawa.

Davis, F. (1976) Who's having the baby – you or the doctor? *Women's Day*, March, **10**, 146–8, 152.

Davis, L. & Riedmann, G. (1990) Recommendations for the management of low risk obstetric patients. *International Journal of Gynecology and Obstetrics*, **35**, 107–15.

Davis-Floyd, R. (1988). Birth as an American rite of passage. In: *Childbirth in America. Anthropological Perspectives*, (ed. Michaelson & Karen), pp. 153–72. Bergin and Garvey, South Hadley, Massachusetts.

DeLee, J. B. (1913) *Principles and Practices of Obstetrics*, 1st edn. W. B. Saunders, Philadelphia.

DeLee, J. B. (1920a) The prophylactic forceps operation. Paper read before the 45th Annual Meeting of the American Gynecological Society, 24–26 May 1920. *American Journal of Obstetrics and Gynecology*, **1**, 24–44, Discussion 77–80.

DeLee, J. B. (1920b) The prophylactic forceps operation. Read before the 45th Annual Meeting of the American Gynecological Society, 24–26 May 1920. *Transactions of the American Gynecology Society*, **45**.

DeLee, J. B. (1921) Discussion of Holmes' paper entitled 'The fads and fancies of obstetrics. A comment on the pseudoscientific trend of modern obstetrics'. Paper read before the Annual Meeting of the American Gynecological Society, Swampscott, Massachusetts, 2–4 June 1921. *American Journal of Obstetrics and Gynecology*, **2** (3), 298–300.

Department of Health, and Office of Population Censuses and Surveys (1988) *Hospital In-patient Enquiry. Maternity Table, England 1982–1985*. HMSO, London.

Department of Health and Social Security, and Office of Population Censuses and Surveys Welsh Office (1986) *Hospital In-patient Enquiry. Maternity Tables, England and Wales 1977–1981*. HMSO, London.

D'Errico, E. & McKeogh, R. (1951) Complete perineotomy. *American Journal of Obstetrics and Gynecology*, **62** (6), 1333–7.

Deutschman, D. (1924) A plea for the preservation of the perineum and a modified prophylactic episiotomy for the prevention of perineal lacerations. Paper read before the Clinical Society of the Bronx Hospital, 8 October 1923 and the Obstetrical and Gynecological Society of the Bronx, January 1924. *Medical Journal and Record*, **120** (19 November), CL–CLIII.

Dewees, W. (1889) Relaxation and management of the perineum during parturition. Paper read before the Golden Belt District Medical Society of Kansas, 4 July 1889. *Journal of the American Medical Association*, **13** (7, 14 December), 804–808, 841–8.

Dewhurst, C. J. (ed.) (1972) *Integrated Obstetrics and Gynaecology for Postgraduates*, 1st edn. Blackwell Scientific Publications, Oxford.

Dewhurst, C. J. (ed.) (1981) *Integrated Obstetrics and Gynaecology for Postgraduates*, 3rd edn. Blackwell Scientific Publications, Oxford.

Dickinson, R. (1920) Suggestions for a program for American gynecology. Address of the President of the American Gynecological Society, Chicago, 24–26 May 1920. *Transactions of the American Gynecological Society*, **45**, 1–13.

Diethelm, M. W. (1938) Episiotomy: technique of repair. Paper read before the Section on Obstetrics and Gynecology, Ohio State Medical Association, 11–12 May 1938. *Ohio State Medical Journal*, **34** (10), 1107–10.

Dixon, A. S. (1990) The evolution of clinical policies. *Medical Care*, **28** (3), 201–220.

Dixon, M. (1981) Episiotomy. Letter to the Editor. *Midwife, Health Visitor and Community Nurse*, **17** (April), 156.

Dobbs, K. & Shy, K. (1981) Alternative birth rooms and birth options. *Obstetrics and Gynecology*, **58** (November), 626–30.

Dodek, S. (1963) Systematic use of muscle relaxants for virtual elimination of rectal involvement with midline episiotomy. *American Journal of Obstetrics and Gynecology*, **87** (2), 272–5.

Doherty, P. & Cohen, I. (1993) Spontaneous vaginal deliveries and perineal trauma in Lucea, Jamaica. *Journal of the Louisiana State Medical Society*, **143** (12), 531–3.

Donald, I. (1955) *Practical Obstetric Problems*, 1st edn. Lloyd-Luke, London.

Donegan, J. (1978) *Women and Men Midwives: Medicine, Morality and Misogyny in Early America*. Greenwood Press, Westport, Connecticut.

Donnison, J. (1977) *Midwives and Medical Men*. Heinemann, London.

Duncan, J. W. (1930) The 'radical' in obstetrics. Paper read before the Brooklyn Gynecological Society, 7 March 1930. *American Journal of Obstetrics and Gynecology*, **20**, 225–35.

Dunn, P. (1985) Galba Araujo of Brazil and episiotomy. Letter to the Editor. *Lancet*, 19 October, 884–5.

Dunne, K. (1984) Characteristics associated with perineal condition in an alternative birth center. *Journal of Nurse-Midwifery*, **29** (January/February), 29–33.

Eastman, N. (1950) *Williams Obstetrics*, 10th edn. Appleton-Century-Crofts, New York.

Eden, T. Watts (1911) *A Manual of Midwifery*, 3rd edn. J. and A. Churchill, London.

Eden, T. Watts (1920) Discussion of DeLee's paper entitled 'The prophylactic forceps operation'. *American Journal of Obstetrics and Gynecology*, **1** (1), 77–8.

Eden, T. Watts & Holland, E. (1937) *A Manual of Obstetrics*, 8th edn. J. & A. Churchill, London.

Edgar, J. Clifton (1903) *The Practice of Obstetrics. Designed for the Use of Students and Practitioners of Medicine*. P. Blackiston's Son and Co., Philadelphia.

Edgar, J. Clifton (1904) The preventive treatment of pelvic floor lacerations. *Transactions of the American Gynecological Society*, **29**, 208–13, 223–32.

Edgar, J. Clifton (1913) *The Practice of Obstetrics. Designed for the Use of Students and Practitioners of Medicine*, 4th edn. P. Blakiston's Son and Co., Philadelphia.

Edwards, M. & Waldorf, M. (1984) *Reclaiming Birth: History and Heroines of American Childbirth Reform*. The Crossing Press, Trumansburg, New York.

Ehrenreich, B. & English, D. (1973) *Witches, Midwives and Nurses: A History of Women Healers*. Glass Mountain Pamphlets, Oyster Bay, New York.

Ehrenreich, B. & English, D. (1979) *For Her Own Good. 150 Years of the Experts' Advice to Women*. Anchor Books, Garden City, New York.

Ehrenreich, J. (ed.) (1978) *The Cultural Crisis in Modern Medicine*. Monthly Review Press, New York.

Eichner, E. (1977) 'Et Tu' Rosemary Cogan and Evelyn Edmunds! Letter to the Editor. *Contemporary OB/GYN*, **10** (November), 16.

Elkin, D. Collier (1922) Median episiotomy. *Journal of the Medical Association of Georgia*, **11**, 224–9.

Elkins, V. Howe (1985) *The Rights of the Pregnant Parent*, revised and updated edn. Lester and Orpen Dennys, Toronto.

Elliott, J. (1978) Letter to the Editor. *Journal of Nurse-Midwifery*, **23** (Spring/Summer), 22–3.

Enkin, M., Hunter, D. J. & Snell, L. (1984) Episiotomy: effects of a research protocol on clinical practice. Editorial. *Birth. Issues in Perinatal Care and Education*, **11** (Autumn), 145–6.

Enkin, M. , Keirse, M. & Chalmers, I. (1989) *A Guide to Effective Care in Pregnancy and Childbirth*. Oxford University Press, New York.

Enkin, M., Keirse, M., Renfrew, M. & Neilson, J. (1995) *A Guide to Effective Care in Pregnancy and Childbirth*, 2nd edn. With the editorial assistance of E. Enkin. Oxford University Press, Oxford.

Everett, H. & Stewart Taylor, E. (1976) The history of the American Gynecological Society and the scientific contributions of its fellows. Paper read before the 99th Annual Meeting of the American Gynecological Society, Hot Springs, Virginia, 25–29 May 1976. *American Journal of Obstetrics and Gynecology*, **127** (7), 908–19.

Farabow, W., Roberson, V., Maxey, J. & Spray, B. (1993) A twenty-year retrospective analysis of the efficacy of epidural analgesia-anesthesia when administered and/or managed by obstetricians. *American Journal of Obstetrics and Gynecology*, **169** (2), 270–78.

Fedrick, J. & Yudkin, P. (1976) Obstetric practice in the Oxford record linkage study area 1965–72. *British Medical Journal*, 27 March, 738–40.

Fernando, B., Leeves, L., Greenacre, J. & Roberts, G. (1995) Audit of the relationship between episiotomy and risk of major perineal laceration during childbirth. *British Journal of Clinical Practice*, **49** (January/February), 40–41.

Finch, J. (1982) Litigation: a simple step forward. *Nursing Mirror*, 8 September.

Finch, J. (1983) Ask mothers first. *Nursing Mirror*, 13 April, 40.

Fischer, S. (1979) Factors associated with the occurrence of perineal lacerations. *Journal of Nurse-Midwifery*, **24** (January/February), 18–26.

Fisher, C. (1981) The management of labour: a midwife's view (ed. S. Kitzinger). In: *Episiotomy: Physical and Emotional Aspects*. National Childbirth Trust, London.

Fleissig, A. (1993) Prevalence of procedures in childbirth. *British Medical Journal*, **306** (20), 494–5.

Flew, J. D. S. (1944) Episiotomy. *British Medical Journal*, 11 November, 620–23.

Flint, C. (1985) Fact-finding mission. Arena. *Nursing Times*, 22 May, 23.

Flint, C. (1986) *Sensitive Midwifery*. Heinemann, London.

Flood, C. (1982) The real reason for performing episiotomies. In Reply. *World Medicine*, 6 February, 51.

Floud, E. (1994a) Protecting the perineum in childbirth 1: a retrospective review. *British Journal of Midwifery*, **2** (June), 258–63.

Floud, E. (1994b) Protecting the perineum in childbirth 2: risk of laceration. *British Journal of Midwifery*, **3** (July), 306–10.

Formato, L.-S. (1985) Routine prophylactic episiotomy. Is it always necessary? *Journal of Nurse-Midwifery*, **30** (May/June), 144–8.

Foss, L. B. (1977) *The incidence of lacerations in nurse-midwife managed deliveries*. Master's thesis, University of Illinois at the Medical Center, Chicago.

Fox, J. S. (1979) Episiotomy. *Midwives Chronicle and Nursing Notes*, October, 337–40.

Fraser, C. (1983) Selected perinatal procedures. Scientific basis for use of psycho-social effects. A literature review. *Acta Obstetricia et Gynecologica Scandinavica*, (117), 5–39.

Freedman, B. (1987) Equipoise and the ethics of clinical research. *New England Journal of Medicine*, **317** (16 July), 141–5.

Friese, K., Labeit, D., Runkel, S. & Meichert, F. (1993) Routine vs. selective episiotomy. Letter to the Editor. *Lancet,* **343** (19 February), 486–7.

Froshaug, J. (1974) The unkindest cut of all? *Nova,* September, 84–5.

Fulsher, R., & Fearl, C. (1955) The third-degree laceration in modern obstetrics. *American Journal of Obstetrics and Gynecology,* **63**, 786–93.

Gainey, H. (1943) Post partum observation of pelvic tissue damage. Paper presented by invitation at the Annual Meeting of the American Association of Obstetricians, Gynecologists and Abdominal Surgeons, 10–12 September 1942. *American Journal of Obstetrics and Gynecology,* **45**, 457–66.

Galabin, A. & Blacker, G. (1910) *The Practice of Midwifery,* 7th edn. The Macmillan Company, New York.

Galloway, C. E. (1935) The management of vertex presentation by episiotomy and forceps. Paper read before the Evanston Branch, Chicago Medical Society. *Illinois Medical Journal,* **67** (June), 536–9.

Garcia, J. & Garforth, S. (1989) Labour and delivery routines in English consultant maternity units. *Midwifery,* **5** 155–62.

Garrey, M. (1982) Episiotomy. Letter to the Editor. *British Medical Journal,* **284** (20 February), 595.

Garrigues, H. J. (1880) The obstetric treatment of the perineum. *American Journal of Obstetrics and Diseases of Women and Children,* **13** (April), 231–63.

Gaskin, I. M. (1977) *Spiritual Midwifery.* The Book Publishing Company, Summertown, Tennessee.

Gass, M. Stopps, Dunn, C. & Stys, S. (1986) Effect of episiotomy on the frequency of vaginal outlet lacerations. *Journal of Reproductive Medicine,* **31**, 240–244.

Gaylin, J. (1982) Sex after childbirth. *Glamour,* **80** (May), 78, 80, 82.

Gerrits, D. D., Brand, R. & Bennebroek Gravenhorst, J. (1994) The use of episiotomy in relation to the professional education of the delivery attendant. *European Journal of Obstetrics and Gynecology,* **56**, 103–106.

Gibberd, G. F. *et al.* (1956) *The Queen Charlotte's Practice of Obstetrics* (9th edn). J. & A. Churchill, London.

Gillespie, C. (1992) *Your Pregnancy Month by Month,* 4th edn. Harper Perennial, New York.

Gillie, O. (1981) Unkind cuts and natural tears. *The Sunday Times,* 20 September, 36.

Gillis, R. A. D. (1930) Episiotomy as a means of preserving the pelvic floor during labor, with a simple method of suture. Presented as a thesis to the Fellows of the American Association of Obstetricians, Gynecologists and Abdominal Surgeons, September 1929. *American Journal of Surgery,* **9** (3), 520–26.

Goodell, W. (1871) A critical inquiry into the management of the perineum during labour. *American Journal of the Medical Sciences,* **61**, 53–79.

Goodlin, R. (1983) On protection of the maternal perineum during birth. *Obstetrics and Gynecology,* **62** (September), 393–4.

Gordon, H. & Logue, M. (1985) Perineal muscle function after childbirth. *Lancet,* 20 July, 123–5.

Graham, H. (1960) *Eternal Eve. The Mysteries of Birth and the Customs that Surround it.* Hutchinson, London.

Graham, H. & Oakley, A. (1981) Competing ideologies of reproduction: medical and maternal perspectives on pregnancy. In: *Women, Health and Reproduction* (ed. H. Roberts). Routledge & Kegan Paul, Boston.

Graham, I. D. (1995) *The episiotomy crusade.* PhD thesis, McGill University, Montreal.

Graham, I. D. (1996) I believe therefore I practice. *Lancet,* **347**, 4–5.

Graham, S. B., Catanzarite, V., Bernstein, J. & Varela-Gittings, F. (1990). A comparison of attitudes and practices of episiotomy among obstetrical practitioners in New Mexico. *Social Science and Medicine,* **31** (2), 191–201.

Green, J. & Soohoo, S. (1989) Factors associated with rectal injury in spontaneous deliveries. *Obstetrics and Gynecology,* **73** (5), 732–8.

Griffiths, M. (1992) Perineal tears. Letter to the Editor. *British Medical Journal,* **305** (12 September), 649.

Gross, S. D. (1884) Laceration of the female sexual organs consequent upon parturition: their causes and their prevention. Paper read before the Section on Obstetrics and Diseases of Women, American Medical Association, May 1884. *Journal of the American Medical Association,* **3** (27 September), 337–45.

Gunn, A. (1967) Episiotomy. *Nursing Times,* **63** (17 March), 342–3.

Gusman, H. A. (1932) The prophylactic use of episiotomy in primipara. Paper read before the Obstetrical and Gynecological Section of the Academy of Medicine of Cleveland, 2 December 1931. *Ohio Medical Journal,* **28** (September), 653–6.

Guyatt, G. H., Sackett, D. L., Cook, D. J. (for the Evidence-Based Medicine Working Group) (1994) Users' guides to the medical literature, II: how to use clinical practice guidelines, B: what were the results and will they help me in caring for my patients? *Journal of the American Medical Association,* **271,** 59–63.

Guyatt, G. H., Sackett, D. L., Sinclair, J., Hayward, R., Cook, D. J. & Cook, R. (for the Evidence-Based Medicine Working Group) (1995) Users' guides to the medical literature, IX: a method for grading health care recommendations. *Journal of the American Medical Association,* **274** (13 December), 1800–1804.

Haigh, A. (1981) Childbirth operation 'ruins sex lives'. *The Times (of London),* 25 September, Home News 3.

Haire, D. B. (1972) *The cultural warping of childbirth.* A special report on US obstetrics prepared for the International Childbirth Education Association, Minneapolis, Minnesota.

Haire, D. B. (1978) The cultural warping of childbirth. In: *The Cultural Crisis of Modern Medicine* (ed. J. Ehrenreich), pp. 185–200. Monthly Review Press, New York.

Hannah, C. R. (1930) Anatomy of the female pelvis and perineum in relation to labor. *American Journal of Obstetrics and Gynecology,* **19,** 228–34.

Harrar, J. (1919a) Median episiotomy in primiparous labors. *Transactions of the American Association of Obstetricians and Gynecologists,* **32,** 117–20, Discussion 120–26.

Harrar, J. (1919b) Median episiotomy in primiparous labors. *American Journal of Obstetrics and Gynecology,* **80,** 705–708.

Harrar, J. (1919c) Median episiotomy in primiparous labors. Paper read before the American Association of Obstetricians and Gynecologists, 15–19 September 1919. *Journal of the American Medical Association,* **23** (25 October), 1307.

Harrar, J. (1923) Functional dystocia in normal pelves: recognition and management. Paper presented at the 35th Annual Meeting of the American Association of Obstetricians, Gynecologists and Abdominal Surgeons, Albany, New York, 19–21 September 1922. *American Journal of Obstetrics and Gynecology,* **15,** 246–94, Discussion 294–7.

Harrison, M. (1982) *A Woman in Residence. A Doctor's Personal and Professional Battles Against an Insensitive Medical System.* Penguin Books, New York.

Harrison, R. F., Brennan, M., North, P. M., Reed, J. V. & Wickham, E. A. (1984) Is routine episiotomy necessary? *British Medical Journal,* **288** (30 June), 1971–5.

Hartko, W. (1978) Letter to the Editor. *Journal of Nurse-Midwifery,* **23** (Spring/Summer), 22–3.

Hayward, R. S. A., Wilson, M. C., Tunis, S. R., Bass, E. B. & Guyatt, G. (for the Evidence-Based Medicine Working Group) (1995) Users' guides to the medical literature, VIII: how to use clinical practice guidelines, A: are the recommendations valid? *Journal of the American Medical Association,* **274** (7), 570–74.

Hazell, L. (1974) *Birth Goes Home.* Catalyst Press, Seattle.

Hazell, L. (1975) A study of 300 elective home births. *Birth and the Family Journal,* **2** (1), 11–23.

Hazell, L. (1976) *Commonsense Childbirth.* Berkley Press, New York.

Helwig, J., Thorp, J. M., Jr & Bowes, W. (1993) Does midline episiotomy increase the risk of third-and fourth-degree lacerations in operative vaginal deliveries? *Obstetrics and Gynecology,* **82** (August), 276–9.

Henriksen, T. Brink, Moller Bek, K., Hedegaard, M. & Secher, N. J. (1992) Episiotomy and perineal lesions in spontaneous vaginal deliveries. *British Journal of Obstetrics and Gynaecology*, **99** (December), 950–54.

Henriksen, T. Brink, Moller Bek, K., Hedegaard, M. & Secher, N. J. (1994) [Episiotomy and perineal lesions in spontaneous vaginal deliveries]. *Ugeskrift for Laeger*, **156** (21), 3176–9.

Henriksen, T. Brink, Moller Bek, K., Hedegaard, M. & Secher, N. J. (1994) Methods and consequences of changes in use of episiotomy. *British Medical Journal*, **309** (12 November), 1255–8.

Hetherington, S. (1990) A controlled study of the effects of prepared childbirth classes on obstetric outcomes. *Birth*, **17** (June), 86–90.

Hillard, P. (1984) Episiotomy. *Parents*, **59** (February), 84, 86.

Hirsch, H. A. (1991) [Pro and Contra Episiotomy]. Editorial. *Gynakologe*, **24** (1), 1–2.

Hirst, Barton Cooke (1902) *A Text-book of Obstetrics*, 3rd edn. W. B. Saunders, Philadelphia.

Hodgkin, R. (1982) Episiotomy. Letter to the Editor. *British Medical Journal*, **284** (3 April), 1042.

Hofmeister, F. (1952) Reconstructive perineal repair of rectovaginal fistulas and injuries occurring at parturition. *American Journal of Surgery*, **84**, 566–73.

Hofmeyr, G. J. & Sonnendecker, E. W. W. (1987) Elective episiotomy in perspective. *South African Medical Journal*, **71**, 357–9.

Holland, E. (1936) Birth injury in relation to labor. Paper presented at the Annual Meeting of the American Gynecological Society, 1936. *Transactions of the American Gynecological Society*, **61**, 47–64.

Holland, E. & Bourne, A. (eds) (1955) *British Obstetric and Gynaecolgical Practice*. William Heinemann, London.

Holmes, R. W. (1921) The fads and fancies of obstetrics. A comment on the pseudo-scientific trend of modern obstetrics. Paper read at the Annual Meeting of the American Gynecological Society, Swampscott, Massachusetts, 2–4 June 1921. *American Journal of Obstetrics and Gynecology*, **2** (3), 225–37, Discussion 297–304.

Homsi, R., Daikoku, N., Littlejohn, J. & Wheeless, C. (1994) Episiotomy: risks of dehiscence and rectovaginal fistula. *Obstetrical and Gynecological Survey*, **49** (12), 803–808.

Hordnes, K. (1994) [Episiotomy – an appeal for a more restricted use]. *Tiddsskrift for Den Norske Laegeforening*, **114** (30), 2641–3642.

House, M. J. (1981a) Episiotomy – indications, technique and results. *Midwife, Health Visitor and Community Nurse*, **17** (January), 6–9.

House, M. H. (1981b) To do or not to do episiotomy? In: *Episiotomy. Physical and Emotional Aspects* (ed. S. Kitzinger), pp. 6–11. National Childbirth Trust, London.

House, M. J., Cario, G. & Jones, M. H. (1986) Episiotomy and the perineum: a random controlled trial. *Journal of Obstetrics and Gynaecology*, **7**, 107–10.

Hughey, M., McElin, T. & Young, T. (1978) Maternal and fetal outcomes of lamaze prepared patients. *Obstetrics and Gynecology*, **51** (6), 643–57.

Hundley, V. A., Cruickshank, F. M., Lang, G. D., Glazener, C. M. A., Milne, J. M., Turner, M., Blyth, D., Mollison, J. & Donaldson, C. (1994) Midwife managed delivery unit: a randomised controlled comparison with consultant led care. *British Medical Journal*, **309** (26 November), 1400–1404.

Hyams, L. (1977) 'Et tu' Rosemary Cogan and Evelyn Edmunds! Letter to the Editor. *Contemporary OB/GYN*, **10** (November), 13, 16.

Inch, S. (1984) *Birthrights. What Every Parent Should Know About Childbirth in Hospitals*, first American edn. Pantheon, New York.

Jackson, M. B. & Dunster, G. D. (1984) Episiotomy: who gets one and why. *Journal of the Royal College of General Practitioners*, November, 603–605.

Jacoby, A. & Cartwright, A. (1990) Finding out about the views and experiences of maternity-service users. In: *The Politics of Maternity Care* (eds J. Garcia, R. Kilpatrick & M. Richards), pp. 238–55. Clarendon Press, Oxford.

Jaeschke, R., Guyatt, G. H. & Sackett, D. L. (for the Evidence-Based Medicine Working Group) (1994a) Users' guides to the medical literature, III: how to use an article about a diagnostic test, A: are the results of the study valid? *Journal of the American Medical Association*, **271** (5), 389–91.

Jaeschke, R., Guyatt, G. H. & Sackett, D. L. (for the Evidence-Based Medicine Working Group) (1994b) Users' guides to the medical literature, III: how to use an article about a diagnostic test, B: what are the results and will they help me in caring for my patient?' *Journal of the American Medical Association*, **271** (9), 703–707.

Jellett, H. (1905) *A Manual of Midwifery for Students and Practitioners*. William Wood and Co., New York.

Jellett, H. & Madill, D. (1929) *A Manual of Midwifery for Students and Practitioners*. Baillière, Tindall and Cox, London.

Jennings, B. (1982) Childbirth choices: are there safe options? *Nurse Practitioner*, July/August, 26–37.

Jewett, C. (1890) Note on Episiotomy. Paper read before the Medical Society of the County of Kings, 17 June 1890. *Brooklyn Medical Journal*, **4**, 707–709.

Johnstone, R. (1913) *A Textbook of Midwifery*. Adam and Charles Black, London.

Kaltreider, D. F. & McClelland Dixon, D. (1948) A study of 710 complete lacerations following central episiotomy. Paper read before the Annual Meeting of the Southern Medical Association, Baltimore, 24–26 November 1947. *Southern Medical Journal*, **41** (9), 814–20.

Katz Rothman, B. (1984) *Giving Birth: Alternatives in Childbirth*. Penguin Books, Harrisonburg, Virginia.

Kaufman, K. & McDonald, H. (1988) A retrospective evaluation of a model of midwifery care. *Birth*, **15** (June), 95–9.

Kaufmann, S. C. (1992) 'To cut or not to cut?' Editorial. *Online Journal of Current Clinical Trials*, 20 August, Doc. No. 16.

Keene, F. E. (ed.) (1930) *Album of the Fellows of the American Gynecological Society 1876–1930*. Wm. J. Dornan, Printer, Philadelphia.

Kelly, R. (1928) The care and repair of the cervix and perineum in confinement cases. Paper read before the Southwestern Virginia Medical Society, 22 September 1927. *Virginia Medical Monthly*, **54** (February), 713–18.

Kelly, R. (1930) Perineotomy versus laceration. Paper read before the Annual Meeting of the Medical Society of Virginia, 22–24 October 1929. *Virginia Medical Record*, **57** (September), 397–400, Discussion 400–401.

Kempster, H. (1986) Guarding the Perineum. *Nursing Times*, 10 September, 51–2.

Kempster, H. (1987) Confused, Battered and Unwanted. *Community Outlook*, June, 8–10.

Kerr, J. M. Munro (1937) *Operative Obstetrics: A Guide to the Difficulties and Complications of Obstetric Practice*, 4th edn. Baillière, Tindall and Cox, London.

Kerr, J. M. Munro & Chassar Moir, J. (1949) *Operative Obstetrics: A Guide to the Difficulties and Complications of Obstetric Practice*, 5th edn. Baillière, Tindall and Cox, London.

Kitzinger, J. (1990) Strategies of the early childbirth movement: a case-study of the national childbirth trust. In: *The Politics of Maternity Care* (eds J. Garia, R. Kilpatrick & M. Richards), pp. 92–115. Clarendon Press, Oxford.

Kitzinger, S. (ed.) (1972) *Episiotomy. Physical and Emotional Aspects*. National Childbirth Trust, London.

Kitzinger, S. (1979a) Episiotomy. Controversy. *Midwife, Health Visitor and Community Nurse*, **15** (6), 233–4.

Kitzinger, S. (1979b) *The Good Birth Guide*. Croom Helm, London.

Kitzinger, S,. (ed.) (1981) *Episiotomy. Physical and Emotional Aspects*, 2nd edn. National Childbirth Trust, London.

Kitzinger, S. (1982) Episiotomy. Letter to the Editor. *British Medical Journal*, **284** (13 March), 823.

Kitzinger, S. (1983) *The New Good Birth Guide*. Penguin Books, London.

Kitzinger, S. (1984) Episiotomy pain. In: *Textbook of Pain* (eds P. Wall & R. Melzack), pp. 293–303. Churchill Livingstone, New York.

Kitzinger, S. (1985) Focusing on today's issues in perinatal care. Episiotomy. *ICEA Review*, **9** (August), 1–7.

Kitzinger, S. (1987) *Your Baby, Your Way*, first American edn. Pantheon, New York.

Kitzinger, S. (1988) *The Complete Book of Pregnancy and Childbirth*, 12th edn. Alfred A. Knopf, New York.

Kitzinger, S. & Simkin, P. (eds) (1984) *Episiotomy and the Second Stage of Labor*. Penny Press, Seattle.

Kitzinger, S. & Simkin, P. (eds) (1986) *Episiotomy and the Second Stage of Labor*, 2nd edn. Penny Press, Seattle.

Kitzinger, S. & Walters, R. (1981) *Some Women's Experiences of Episiotomy*. National Childbirth Trust, London.

Klein, M. (1988) Rites of passage: episiotomy and the second stage of labour. *Canadian Family Physician*, **34** (September), 2019–25.

Klein, M., Gauthier, R., Jorgenson, S., *et al.* (1992) Does episiotomy prevent perineal trauma and pelvic floor relaxation? *Online Journal of Current Clinical Trials*, **1** July, Doc. No. 10.

Klein, M., Gauthier, R., Robbins, J., *et al.* (1994) Relationship of episiotomy to perineal trauma and morbidity, sexual dysfunction, and pelvic floor relaxation. *American Journal of Obstetrics and Gynecology*, **171** (September), 591–8.

Klein, M., Kaczoworwski, J., Robbins, J., *et al.* (1995) Physicians' beliefs and behaviour during a randomized controlled trial of episiotomy: consequences for women in their care. *Canadian Medical Association Journal*, **153** (6) (15 September), 796–9.

Korbin, F. (1966) The American midwife controversy: a crisis in professionalization. *Bulletin of the History of Medicine*, **40**, 350–63.

Korte, D. & Scaer, R. (1990) *A Good Birth, a Safe Birth*, revised & expanded edn. Bantam Books, New York.

Kozak, L. (1989) Surgical and nonsurgical procedures associated with hospital delivery in the United States: 1980–1987. *Birth*, **16** (December), 209–13.

Kretzschmar, N. R. & Huber, C. P. (1938) A study of 2 987 consecutive episiotomies. *American Journal of Obstetrics and Gynecology*, **35** (4), 621–6.

Kuller, J. A., Wells, S. R., Thorp, J. M., Jr & Bowes, W. A. (1994) Obstetric damage and faecal incontinence. *Lancet*, **344** (19 November), 1435.

Läärä, E. (1984) Is routine episiotomy necessary? Letter to the Editor. *British Medical Journal*, **289** (8 September), 627.

Lake, A. (1976) Childbirth in America. *McCall's*, January, 83, 128–30, 142.

Larsson, Per-Göran, Jens-Jörgen, *et al.* (1991) Advantage or disadvantage of episiotomy compared with spontaneous perineal laceration. *Gynecology and Obstetric Investigations*, **31**, 213–16.

Lau, Y. K. (1982) How women view postepisiotomy pain. Letter to the Editor. *British Medical Journal*, **284** (3 April), 1041–2.

Laupacis, A., Wells, G., Richardson, W. S. & Tugwell, P. (for the Evidence-Based Medicine Working Group) (1994) Users' guides to the medical literature, V: how to use an article about prognosis. *Journal of the American Medical Association*, **272** (3), 234–7.

Leavitt, J. Walzer (1983) 'Science' enters the birthing room. Obstetrics in America since the eighteenth century. *Journal of American History*, **70** (2), 281–304.

Leavitt, J. Walzer (1986) *Brought to Bed: Childbearing in America 1750–1950*. Oxford University Press, New York.

Lee, B. (1982) Episiotomy. Letter to the Editor. *British Medical Journal*, **284** (20 February), 595.

Levett, D. (1974) Episiotomy – an over-used procedure? Open Forum. *Nursing Mirror*, 17 October, 89.

Lewis, L. S. (1984) West Berkshire perineal management trial. Letter to the Editor. *British Medical Journal*, **289** (29 September), 837.

Lieberman, A. (1989) Must you have an episiotomy? *American Baby*, **51** (February), 51.

Llewellyn-Jones, J. D. (1987) Letter to the Editor. *British Journal of Obstetrics and Gynaecology*, **94** (January), 92.

Logue, M. (1991) Putting research into practice: perineal management during delivery. In: *Midwives, Research and Childbirth* (S. Robinson & A. Thomson), pp. 252–70. Chapman and Hall, London.

Longo, L. D. (1976) Rigidity of soft parts. Delivery effected by incision on the perineum. *Obstetrics and Gynecology*, **25** (1 May), 115.

Longo, M. (1989) Why cut? *Great Expectations*, April, 40–42.

Lubin, S. (1932) Episiotomy versus laceration. *Medical Times and Long Island Medical Journal*, **60** (March), 8283.

Lusk, W. Thompson (1884) *The Science and Art of Midwifery*. D. Appleton and Co., New York.

Lynch, F. (1924) The speciality of gynecology and obstetrics. Chairman's Address to the Section on Obstetrics, Gynecology and Abdominal Surgery, American Medical Association, Chicago, June 1924. *Journal of the American Medical Association*, **83** (9 August), 397–9.

Lydon-Rochelle, M., Albers, L. & Teaf, D. (1995) Perineal outcomes and nurse-midwifery management. *Journal of Nurse-Midwifery*, **40** (1), 13–18.

MacCallum, L. (1982) The episiotomy: what it is; can you avoid one? *Glamour* **80** (October), 172.

McCausland, A. M. (1938) Discussion of Huff's paper entitled 'Mediolateral episiotomy'. *California and Western Medicine*, **48** (March), 178–9.

McCormick, F. & Renfrew, M. (1996) *The Midwifery Research Database. A Source Book of Information About Research in Midwifery*, 2nd edn. Books for Midwives Press, Hale, Cheshire.

McCullough, A. M. (1984) Episiotomy. *Journal of the Royal Army Medical Corps*, **130** (1), 60–63.

Macfarlane, A. & Mugford, M. (1984). *Birth Counts. Statistics of Pregnancy and Childbirth*. Her Majesty's Stationery Office, London.

McGuinness, M., Norr, K. & Nacion, K. (1991) Comparison between different perineal outcomes on tissue healing. *Journal of Nurse-Midwifery*, **36** (3), 192–8.

McKinlay, J. B. (1981) From 'promising report' to 'standard procedure': seven stages in the career of a medical innovation. *Milbank Memorial Fund Quarterly/Health and Society*, **59** (3), 374–411.

MacLennan, A. H. (1978) An audit of obstetric practice in the management of labour. *Australian and New Zealand Journal of Obstetrics and Gynecology*, **18**, 287–8.

MacLennan, A. H. (1990) Perineal pain after childbirth. Leading article. *Medical Journal of Australia*, **152**, 1–2.

Madden, T. More (1872) On lacerations of the perinaeum, sphincter ani, and recto-vaginal septum – their prevention and surgical treatment. *American Journal of Obstetrics and Diseases of Women and Children*, **5**, 50–78.

Manton, W. P. (1885) A plea for episiotomy. *American Journal of Obstetrics and Diseases of Women and Children*, **28** (March), 225–35.

Martin, E. (1989) *The Woman in the Body: A Cultural Analysis of Reproduction*. Beacon Press, Boston.

Massey, G. & Bates, R. (1975) Letter to the Editor. *British Journal of Medicine*, 29 March, 732–3.

Maves, H. M. (1987) Management of the second stage. *Midwife, Health Visitor and Community Nurse*, **23** (11), 498, 502–506.

Maxwell, J. (1986) The iron lung: halfway technology or necessary step? *Milbank Quarterly*, **64** (1), 3–29.

Maynard, F. (1977) Home births vs. hospital births. *Women's Day*, 28 June, 10, 12, 161–2, 164.

Mazzarella, G., Scarpellino, B., Coppola, A., Cafiero, M., Quagiata, L. & Pisacane, A. (1991) Antenatal and perinatal care in southern Italy. II. The clinicians' reactions. *Paediatric and Perinatal Epidemiology*, **5** (1), 78–82.

Mehl, L. (1977) Outcomes of elective home births: a series of 1146 cases. *Journal of Reproductive Medicine*, **19**, 281–90.

Mehl, L. (1977–78) Options in maternity carer. *Women and Health,* **2–3**, 29–42.

Mehl, L. (1978a) The outcome of home delivery in the United States. In: *The Place of Birth* (eds S. Kitzinger & J. Davis), pp. 107. Oxford University Press, New York.

Mehl, L. (1978b) Scientific research on childbirth alternatives: what can it tell us about hospital practice? In: *21st Century Obstetrics Now! Vol. 1* (eds L. Stewart & D. Stewart), pp. 171–208. NAPSAC, Marble Hill, Missouri.

Miller, R. (1960) An analysis of generalists' obstetrics. *American Journal of Obstetrics and Gynecology,* **80** (4), 813–22.

Moir, J. Chassar & Myerscough, P. R. (1971) *Munro Kerr's Operative Obstetrics.* 8th edn. Baillière, Tindall and Cox, London.

Morris, N. (1981) A very common operation. Editorial. *Midwife, Health Visitor and Community Nurse,* **17** (January), 3.

Morris, W. I. C. (1974) Pain after Birth. Letter to the Editor. *British Medical Journal,* **901** (9 February), 243.

Morton, L. T. (1954) *Garrison and Morton's Medical Directory: An Annotated Check-list of Texts Illustrating the History of Medicine,* 2nd edn. Grafton and Co., London.

Moses, F. (1992) Episiotomy vs. perineal tear: which is less traumatic? *British Journal of Nursing,* **1** (15), 758–61.

Murphy-Black, T. (1993) Research and the midwife. In: *Myles Textbook For Midwives* (eds V. R. Bennett & L. K. Brown), pp. 770–80. Churchill Livingstone, London.

National Center for Health Statistics (1992) *Vital and Health Statistics. National Hospital Discharge Survey: Annual Summary, 1990.* US Department of Health and Human Services. Public Health Service. Centers for Disease Control, Hyattsville, Maryland. DHHS Publication No. (HPS) 91–1773.

National Center for Health Statistics (1993) *Vital and Health Statistics. National Hospital Discharge Survey: Annual Summary, 1991.* US Department of Health and Human Services. Public Health Service. Centers for Disease Control, Hyattsville, Maryland. DHHS Publication No. (HPS) 91–1775.

National Center for Health Statistics (1994) *Vital and Health Statistics. National Hospital Discharge Survey: Annual Summary, 1992.* US Department of Health and Human Services. Public Health Service. Centers for Disease Control, Hyattsville, Maryland. DHHS Publication No. (HPS) 94–1779.

National Center for Health Statistics (1995) *Vital and Health Statistics. National Hospital Discharge Survey: Annual Summary, 1993.* US Department of Health and Human Services, Public Health Service, Centers for Disease Control, DHHS Publication No. (HPS) 95–1782.

National Student Nurses Association (1979) Episiotomy as an American Phenomenon. Resolution passed by the National Student Nurses Association, St Louis, Missouri, 22–30 April 1978. *Journal of Nurse-Midwives,* **24** (1), 31.

Naugle, D., Sorenson, R. & Kiser, W. (1994) Letter to the Editor. *Lancet,* **343**, 486–7.

Naylor, C. D. & Guyatt, G. H. (for the Evidence-Based Medicine Working Group) (1996) Users' guides to the medical literature, XI: how to use an article about clinical utilization review. *Journal of the American Medical Association,* **275** (18), 1435–9.

Naylor, C. D. & Guyatt, G. H. (for the Evidence-Based Medicine Working Group) (in press) Users' guides to the medical literature, X: how to use an article reporting variations in the outcomes of health services. *Journal of the American Medical Association.*

Neal, E. Jewel (1923) Sane obstetrics. Paper read before the State Society of Iowa Medical Women, Ottumwa, Iowa, 8 May 1923. *Medical Woman's Journal,* 30 October, 289–92.

Needham, D. & Sheriff, J. (1983) A survey on tears and episiotomies of the perineum. *Midwife, Health Visitor and Community Nurse,* **96** (July), 232–3.

Nelson, H. Bristol & Abramson, D. (1941) The advantages of conservative obstetrics as shown by examination six weeks post partum. Paper read before the Obstetrical Society of Boston, 28 February 1941. *American Journal of Obstetrics and Gynecology,* **52**, 800–811.

Neville-Smith, C. H. (1984) How informed are patients who have given informed consent? Letter to the Editor. *British Medical Journal*, **289** (1 September), 837.

Newton, M. (1977) The 'most unkindest cut' indeed, agrees Professor. Letter to the Editor. *Contemporary OB/GYN*, **10** (November), 13.

Nodine, P. & Roberts, J. (1987) Factors associated with perineal outcome during childbirth. *Journal of Nurse-Midwifery*, **32** (May/June), 123–30.

Norwood, C. (1978) A humanizing way to have a baby. *Ms*, **6** (May), 89–92.

Nugent, F. (1935) The primiparous perineum after forceps delivery. Paper presented to the Obstetrical Society of Philadelphia. *American Journal of Obstetrics and Gynecology*, **30**, 249–56.

Oakley, A. (1976) *Wise women and medicine men: changes in the management of childbirth* (eds J. Mitchell & A. Oakley). In: *The Rights and Wrongs of Women*. Penguin, Harmondsworth.

Oakley, A. (1979) *Becoming a Mother*. Martin Robertson, Oxford.

Oakley, A. (1986) *The Captured Womb: a History of the Medical Care of Pregnant Women*. Basil Blackwell, New York.

O'Driscoll, K. & Meagher, D. (1980) *The Active Management of Labour*. Baillière, Tindall and Cox, London.

O'Driscoll, K., Stronge, J. M. & Minogue, M. (1973) Active management of labour. *British Medical Journal*, **3**, 133–5.

O'Leary, J. L. & O'Leary, J. A. (1965) The complete episiotomy. Analysis of 1224 complete lacerations, sphincterotomies, and episiproctotomies. *Obstetrics and Gynecology*, **25** (2), 235–40.

Olson, R., Olson, C. & Smith Cox, N. (1990) Maternal birthing positions and perineal injury. *Journal of Family Practice*, **30** (5), 553–7.

Oxman, A. D., Sackett, D. L. & Guyatt, G. H. (for the Evidence-Based Medicine Working Group) (1993) Users' guides to the medical literature, I: how to get started. *Journal of the American Medical Association*, **270** (17), 2093–5.

Oxman, A. D., Cook, D. J., Guyatt, G. H. (for the Evidence-Based Medicine Working Group) (1994) Users' guides to the medical literature, VI: how to use an overview. *Journal of the American Medical Association*, **272**, 1367–71.

Paciornik, M. (1990) Commentary: arguments against episiotomy and in favor of squatting position. *Birth*, **17** (June), 104–105.

Pallen, A. Montrose (1876) Perineal lacerations. Paper read before the New York Medical Journal Association, 22 March 1876. *New York Medical Journal*, **23**, 466–79.

Pallet, C. (1977) Some mothers' thoughts on episiotomy, as requested by AIMS in *Mother and Baby* magazine. *AIMS Quarterly Newsletter*, October, 2–4.

Panter, G. (1980) Episiotomy: the question of informed consent. *Parents*, May, 86, 88.

Papst, A. (1982) Letter to the Editor. *Birth. Issues in Perinatal Care and Education*, **9** (Winter), 267–8.

Park, R. E. (1955) *Society: The Collected Papers of Robert Ezra Park*, Vol. 3. The Free Press, Glencoe, Illinois.

Parks, J. & Barter, R. (1954) Operative obstetrics. Paper read before the Washington State Obstetrical Association, 17 October 1953. *Western Journal of Surgery, Obstetrics and Gynecology*, **62** (February), 61–5.

Parvin, T. (1882) Care of the perineum. *Transactions of the American Gynecological Society*, **7**, 145–54, Discussion 154–7.

Parvin, T. (1890) *The Science and Art of Obstetrics*, 2nd edn. Lea Brothers and Co., Philadelphia.

Parvin, T. (1895) *The Science and Art of Obstetrics*, 3rd edn. Lea Brothers and Co., Philadelphia.

Pascoe, E. (1977) How women want to have their babies. *McCall's Monthly Newsletter for Women Right Now*, **105** (October), 109–10.

Paterson-Brown, S., Fisk, N. & Wyatt, J. (1995) Uptake of meta-analytical overviews of effectiveness care in English obstetric units. *British Journal of Obstetrics and Gynaecology*, **102**, 297–301.

Phillips, A. (1978) Letter to the Editor. *Journal of Nurse-Midwifery,* **23** (Spring/Summer), 22.

Pieri, R. J. (1938) The female perineum. Episiotomy and a technic for its repair. *Journal of the American Medical Association,* **110** (21 May), 1738–43.

Pilkington, J., Cunningham, C. & Johnson, R. (1963) Median episiotomy and complete perineotomy. Paper read before the Section on Obstetrics, Southern Medical Association, 6–9 November 1961. *Southern Medical Journal,* **56** (March), 284–6.

Piper, D. & McDonald, P. (1994) Management of anticipated and actual shoulder dystocia. *Journal of Nurse-Midwifery,* **39** (91S–105S).

Playfair, W. Smoults (1882) *A Treatise on the Science and Art of Midwifery,* 4th edn. Smith Elder, London.

Playfair, W. Smoults (1885) *A Treatise on the Science and Art of Midwifery,* 5th edn. Smith Elder, London.

Playfair, W. Smoults (1889) *A Treatise on the Science and Art of Midwifery,* 6th edn. Smith Elder, London.

Playfair, W. Smoults (1898) *A Treatise on the Science and Art of Midwifery.* Smith Elder, London.

Pogmore, R. (1974) Pain after birth. Letter to the Editor. *British Medical Journal,* **895** (5 January), 37.

Polden, M. (1982) Episiotomy. Letter to the Editor. *British Medical Journal,* **284** (13 March), 823.

Polit, D. F. & Hungler, B. (1995) *Nursing Research: Principles and Methods,* 5th edn. Lippincott, Philadelphia.

Pomeroy, R. H. (1918a) Shall we cut and reconstruct the perineum for every primipara? Paper read before the American Gynecological Society, 16–18 May 1918. *American Journal of Obstetrics and Diseases of Women and Children,* **78,** 211–20, Discussion 295–7.

Pomeroy, R. H. (1918b) Shall we cut and reconstruct the perineum for every primipara? *Transactions of the American Gynecological Society,* **43,** 201–206, Discussion 207–12.

Pomeroy, R. H. (1921) Discussion of Holmes' paper entitled 'The fads and fancies of obstetrics'. A comment on the pseudoscientific trend of modern obstetrics. Paper read at the Annual Meeting of the American Gynecological Society, Swampscott, Massachusetts, 2–4 June 1921. *American Journal of Obstetrics and Gynecology,* **2** (3), 300–301.

Presl, J. (1985) [Episiotomy and perineal protection – generally an unnecessary operation and a useless, occasionally risky manoeuvre]. *Ceckoslovenska Gynekologie,* **50** (June), 380–82.

Pretorius, G. P. (1982) Episiotomy. Letter to the Editor. *British Medical Journal,* **284** (1 May), 1332.

Pritchard, J. & MacDonald, P. (1980) *Williams Obstetrics,* 16th edn. Appleton-Century-Crofts, New York.

Pritchard, J., Macdonald P. R. & Gant, N. (1985) *Williams Obstetrics,* 17th edn. Appleton-Century-Crofts, Norwalk, Connecticut.

Quigley, J. (1923) Discussion of Harrar's paper entitled 'Functional dystocia in normal pelves: recognition and management'. *American Journal of Obstetrics and Gynecology,* **15,** 294–5.

Ramin, S. & Gilstrap, L. C. III (1994) Episiotomy and early repair of dehiscence. *Clinical Obstetrics and Gynecology,* **37** (4), 816–23.

Randal, J. (1979) Where should your child be born? *Parents,* March, 74–8.

Ratner, H. (1978) History of the dehumanization of American obstetrical practice. In: *21st Century Obstetrics Now! Vol. 1* (eds L. Stewart & D. Stewart), pp. 115–46. NAPSAC, Marble Hill, Missouri.

Reading, A. E. (1982) How women view postepisiotomy pain. Letter to the Editor. *British Medical Journal,* **284** (3 April), 1042.

Reading, A. E., Sledmere, C. M., Cox, D. N. & Campbell, S. (1982) How women view post episiotomy pain. *British Medical Journal,* **284** (23 January), 243–6.

Reamy, K. & White, S. (1985) Sexuality in pregnancy and the puerperium: a review. *Obstetrical and Gynecological Survey,* **40** (1), 1–13.

Reamy, K. & White, S. (1987) Sexuality in pregnancy and the puerperium: a review. *Archives of Sexual Behavior*, **16** (2), 165–86.

Reamy, T. (1885) Protection of the perineum during parturition. *Transactions of the American Gynecological Society*, **10**, 147–60, 161–71.

Renfrew, M., Fisher, C. & Arms, S. (1990) *Breastfeeding: Getting Breastfeeding Right for You.* Celestial Arts, Berkeley, California.

Reynolds, J. (1993) The final fatal blow to routine episiotomy. Commentary. *Birth*, **20** (September), 162–3.

Reynolds, J. (1995) Reducing the frequency of episiotomies through a continuous quality improvement program. *Canadian Medical Association Journal*, **153** (1 August), 275–364.

Reynolds, J. L. & Yudkin, P. L. (1987) Changes in the management of labour: 2. Perineal management. *Canadian Medical Association Journal*, **136** (15 May), 1045–9.

Richards, M. P. M. (1975) Innovation in medical practice: obstetricians and the induction of labour in Britain. *Social Science and Medicine*, **9** 595–602.

Richardson, W. S. & Detsky, A. S. (for the Evidence-Based Medicine Working Group) (1955a) Users' guides to the medical literature, VII: how to use a clinical decision analysis, A: are the results of the study valid? *Journal of the American Medical Association*, **273** (16), 1292–5.

Richardson, W. S. & Detsky, A. S. (for the Evidence-Based Medicine Working Group) (1995b) Users' guides to the medical literature, VII: how to use a clinical decision analysis, B: what are the results and will they help me in caring for my patients? *Journal of the American Medical Association*, **273** (20), 1610–13.

Roberts, J. & Mokos Kritz, D. (1984). Delivery positions and perineal outcome. *Journal of Nurse-Midwifery*, **29** (May/June), 186–90.

Robinson, J. (1982) The maternity defence complaints confined to childbirth. *Nursing Mirror*, 8 September.

Robinson, S. (1990) Maintaining the independence of the midwifery profession: a continuing struggle. In: *The Politics of Maternity Care* (eds J. Garcia, R. Kilpatrick & M. Richards), pp. 61–91. Clarendon Press, Oxford.

Robinson, S., Golden, J. & Bradley, S. (1983) *A Study of the Role and Responsibilities of the Midwife.* Nursing Education Research Unit, Department of Nursing Studies, Chelsea College, University of London.

Röckner, G. (1993) [Reconsideration of the use of episiotomy in primiparas] *Jordemodern*, **106** (10), 373–5.

Röckner, G. & Olund, A. (1991) The use of episiotomy in primiparas in Sweden. A descriptive study with particular focus on two hospitals. *Acta Obstetricia et Gynecologica Scandinavica*, **70** (4–5), 325–30.

Röckner, G., Wahlberg, V. & Olund, A. (1989) Episiotomy and perineal trauma during childbirth. *Journal of Advanced Nursing*, **14** (April), 264–8.

Romalis, S. (ed.) (1981) *Childbirth: Alternatives to Medical Control.* University of Texas Press, Austin, Texas.

Rosengren, W. & Sartell, K. L. (1986) Current obstetrical technologies: a clash of values. In: *The Adoption and Social Consequences of Medical Technologies* (eds J. Roth & S. Burt Ruzek), pp. 93–146. Research in Sociology of Health Care – A Research Annual, Vol. 4. JAI Press, Greenwich, Connecticut.

Rothschild, C. J. (1915) Episiotomy, a perineal safety measure. Paper read before the Fort Wayne Medical Society, 27 April 1915. *Journal of the Indiana Medical Society*, **8** (September), 416–18.

Ruby, G., Banta, D. & Kesselamn Burns, A. (1984) Medicare coverage, medicare costs, and medical technology. *Journal of Health Politics, Policy and Law*, **10**, 141–55.

Rumeau-Rouguette, C., du Mazanbrun, C. & Rabarison, Y. (1984) *Naître en France. 10 ans d'evolution 1972–1981.* INSERM/DOIN, Paris.

Russell, J. K. (1982) Episiotomy. Editorial. *British Medical Journal*, **284** (23 January), 220.

Ruzek, S. Burt (1978) *The Women's Health Movement.* Praeger Publishers, New York.

Salmond, M. & Dearnley, G. (1935) The prevention of prolapse of the uterus and vaginal walls following childbirth. *Journal of Obstetrics and Gynaecology of the British Empire*, **42**, 446–75.

Savage, J. E. (1957) Lacerations of the birth canal. *Journal of the Louisiana Medical Society*, **109**, 164–72.

Shooirer, M. A. (1990) The life cycle of an innovation: adoption versus discontinuation of the fluoride mouth rinse program in schools. *Journal of Health and Social Behavior*, **31** (June), 203–15.

Schmidt, J. E. (1959) *Medical Discoveries: Who and When.* Thomas, Springfield, Illinois.

Schneider, G. (1981) Management of normal labour and delivery in the case room: a critical appraisal. *Canadian Medical Association Journal*, **125** (15 August), 350–52.

Scholten, C. (1977) On the importance of obstetric art: changing customs of childbirth in America 1870–1815. *William and Mary Quarterly*, **34** (3 July), 426–45.

Scholten, C. (1985) *Childbearing in American Society, 1650-1850.* New York University Press, New York.

Schrag, K. (1979) Maintenance of the pelvic floor integrity during childbirth. *Journal of Nurse-Midwifery*, **24** (November/December), 26–31.

Sellers, T. B. & Sanders J. T. (1930) The prevention and management of birth canal injuries and the anatomical repair of old lacerations of the perineum. Paper read before the Orleans Parish Medical Society. *New Orleans Medical and Surgical Society*, **83**, 757–65.

Shea, P. (1985) Episiotomy, to cut or not to cut: that is the question! *Great Expectations*, October, 19–20.

Shiono, P., Klebanoff, M. & Carey, J. C. (1990) Midline episiotomies: more harm than good? *Obstetrics and Gynecology*, **75** (May), 765–70.

Shorter, E. (1900) *Women's Bodies. A Social History of Women's Encounters with Ill-health, and Medicine.* Transaction Publishers, New Brunswick.

Shorter, E. (1982) *A History of Women's Bodies.* Basic Books, New York.

Shy, K.. & Eschenbach, D. (1979) Fatal perineal cellulitis from an episiotomy site. *Obstetrics and Gynecology*, **54** (3), 292–8.

Sieber, E. H. & Kroon, J. D. (1962) Morbidity in the third-degree laceration. *Obstetrics and Gynecology*, **19** (5), 677–80.

Simkin, P. (1986) Introduction. In: *Episiotomy and the Second Stage of Labour* (eds S. Kitzinger & P. Simkin), pp. 3–5. Penny Press, Seattle.

Simms, C., McHaffie, H., Renfrew, M. & Ashurst, H. (1994) *The Midwifery Research Database. A Source Book of Information About Research in Midwifery.* Books for Midwives Press, Hale, Cheshire.

Simpson, D. (1988) Examining the episiotomy argument. *Midwife, Health Visitor and Community Nurse*, **24** (1), 6–14.

Simpson, J. Young (1871) *Selected Obstetrical and Gynaecological Works of Sir James Y. Simpson. Volume 1.* (ed. J. Watt Black). Adam and Charles Churchill, Edinburgh.

Sisk, J. E. (1993) Improving the use of research-based evidence in policy making: effective care in pregnancy and childbirth in the United States. *Milbank Quarterly*, **71** (477–96).

Skoner, M., Thompson, D. & Caron, V. (1994) Factors associated with risk of stress urinary incontinence in women. *Nursing Research*, **43** (5), 301–306.

Sleep, J. (1984a) Episiotomy in normal delivery. *Nursing*, **2** (January), 614.

Sleep, J. (1984b) Episiotomy in normal delivery. One. *Nursing Times*, 21 November, 29–30.

Sleep, J. (1984c) Episiotomy in normal delivery. Two – Management of the perineum. *Nursing Times*, 28 November, 51–4.

Sleep, J. (1985) [Episiotomy in normal delivery]. *Josanpu Zasshi*, **39** (6), 516–22.

Sleep, J. (1987) Perineal management – a midwifery skill under threat. *Midwife, Health Visitor and Community Nurse*, **23** (20), 455–8.

Sleep, J. (1989) Physiology and management of the second stage of labour. In: *Myles Textbook for Midwives* (eds V. R. Bennett & L. K. Brown), 11th edn., pp. 192–208. Churchill Livingstone, Edinburgh.

Sleep, J. (1993) Physiology and management of the second stage of labour. In *Myles Textbook for Midwives* (eds V. R. Bennett & L. K. Brown), 12th edn., pp. 199–215. Edinburgh: Churchill Livingstone.

Sleep, J. & Grant, A. (1987) West Berkshire perineal management trial: three year follow up. *British Medical Journal*, **295** (26 September), 749–51.

Sleep, J., Grant, A., Garcia, J., Elbourne, D., Spencer, J. & Chalmers, I. (1984) West Berkshire perineal management trial. *British Medical Journal*, **289** (8 September), 587–90.

Sleep, J., Roberts J. & Chalmers, I. (1989) Care during the second stage of labour. In: *Effective Care in Pregnancy and Childbirth* (eds I. Chalmers, M. Enkins & M. Keirse), pp. 1136–44. Oxford University Press, Oxford.

Smith, M., Acheson, L., Byrd, J. *et al.* (1991) A critical review of labor and birth care. *Journal of Family Practice*, **33** (3), 281–92.

Smith, M., Ruffin, M. & Green, L. (1993) The rational management of labor. *American Family Physician*, **47** (1 May), 1471–81.

Smith, S. (1951) The median episiotomy. Its technic and a review of 1500 consecutive cases. Paper read before the Los Angeles Obstetrical and Gynecological Society, Los Angeles, 11 October 1949. *Western Journal of Surgery, Obstetrics and Gynecology*, **59** (March), 102–109.

Spector, M. (1976) The social construction of social problems. *Teaching Sociology*, **3** (2), 167–84.

Spector, M. & Kitsuse, J. (1977) *Constructing Social Problems*. Cummings Publishing Co., Don Mills, Ontario.

Speert, H. (1980) *Obstetric and Gynecology in America: A History*. American College of Obstetrics and Gynecology, Chicago.

Stahl, F. (1895) Concerning the principles and practice of episiotomy – why central preferable to lateral. *Annals of Gynaecology and Paediatry*, **8**, 674–7.

Stewart, L. & Stewart, D. (eds) (1978) *21st Century Obstetrics Now! Volume 1*, pp. 115–46. NAPSAC, Marble Hill, Missouri.

Stiles, D. (1980) Techniques for reducing the need for an episiotomy. *Issues in Health Care of Women*, **2**, 105–111.

Stones, R. W., Paterson, C. M. & Saunders, N. J. (1993) Risk factors for major obstetric haemorrhage. *European Journal of Obstetrics, Gynecology, and Reproductive Biology*, **48** (1), 15–18.

Stratton, J., Gordon, H. & Logue, M. (1995) Conclusions and validity of data cannot be judged. *British Medical Journal*, **310** (11 March), 668.

Sultan, A. H., Kamm, M. A., Hudson, C. N. & Bartram, C. I. (1994) Third degree obstetric anal sphincter tears: risk factors and outcomes of primary repair. *British Medical Journal*, **308** (2 April), 877–91.

Summey, P. & Hurst, M. (1986) Ob/gyn on the rise: the evolution of professional ideology in the twentieth century – Part I. *Women and Health*, **11** (Spring), 133–45.

Task force on the Implementation of Midwifery in Ontario (1987) *Report of the task force on the implementation of midwifery in Ontario*. Government of Ontario Book Store, Toronto.

Taylor, E. S. (1982) Editorial note. *Obstetrical and Gynecological Survey*, **37** (10), 614.

Taylor, E. S. (1986) Editorial note. *Obstetrical and Gynecological Survey*, **41** (4), 230–231.

Taylor, E. S. (1987) Editorial note. *Obstetrical and Gynecological Survey*, **42** (3), 164–5.

Taylor, H. C., Jr (1937) Indications and technique of episiotomy. *American Journal of Surgery*, **35** (2), 403–408.

Thacker, S. & Banta, H. D. (1982) Benefits and risks of episiotomy. *Women and Health*, **7** (3–4), 161–77.

Thacker, S. & Banta, H. D. (1983) Benefits and risks of episiotomy: an interpretative review of the English language literature, 1860–1980. *Obstetrical and Gynecological Survey*, **38** (June), 322–38.

Thompson, D. J. (1987) No episiotomy? *Australian and New Zealand Journal of Obstetrics and Gynaecology*, **27** (1), 18–20.

Thoms, H. (1935) *Classical Contributions to Obstetrics and Gynecology*. Charles C. Thomas, Baltimore.

Thorp, J. & Bowes, W. (1989) Episiotomy: can its routine use be defended? *American Journal of Obstetrics and Gynecology*, **160** (May), 1027–30.

Thorp, J. & Bowes, W. (1991) Reply to Letter to the Editor. *American Journal of Obstetrics and Gynecology*, **164** (3), 936.

Thorp, J., Bowes, W., Brame, R. & Cefalo, R. (1987) Selected use of midline episiotomy: effect on perineal trauma. *Obstetrics and Gynecology*, **70** (August), 260–62.

Thranov, I., Kringekbach, A. M., Melchoir, E., Olson, O. & Damsgaard, M. T. (1990) Postpartum symptoms. Episiotmy or tear at vaginal delivery. *Acta Obstetricia et Gynecologica Scandinavica*, **69** (1), 11–15.

Toal, J. (1986) Episiotomy: do you have a choice? *American Baby*, **48** (September), 41.

Trevelyan, J. (1994) Please tell mother. *Nursing Times*, **90** (9), 38–9.

Triphen, E. R. (1983) *Delivery position and the effect of perineal integrity*. Master's thesis, St Louis University, St Louis, Missouri.

Tritsch, J. E. (1930) Another plea for the prophylactic median episiotomy. *Journal of the American Institute of Homeopathy*, **23**, 327–33.

United States Congress, Office of Technology Assessment (1976) *Development of Medical Technology. Opportunities for Assessment*. US Government Printing Office, Washington DC.

United States Department of Health, Education and Welfare (1976a) *Report of the President's Biomedical Research Panel*. DHEW Publication No. (OS) 76–500.

United States Department of Health, Education and Welfare (1976b) *Report of the President's Biomedical Research Panel. Appendix B. Approaches to Policy Development for Biomedical Research: Strategy for Budgeting and Movement from Invention to Clinical Application*. DHEW Publication No. (OS) 76–502.

Valenstein, E. S. (1986) *Great and Desperate Cures. The Rise and Decline of Psychosurgery and Other Radical Treatments for Mental Illness*. Basic Books, New York.

Van de Warker, E. (1904) Discussion of the symposium on injuries of the perineum, American Gynecological Society, 1904. *Transactions of the American Gynecological Society*, **29**, 226–8.

Varner, M. (1986) Episiotomy: techniques and indications. *Clinical Obstetrics and Gynecology*, **29** (2), 309–17.

Viktrup, L., Lose, G., Rolff, M. & Barfoed, K. (1992) The symptom of stress incontinence caused by pregnancy or delivery in primiparas. *Obstetrics and Gynecology*, **79** (June), 945–9.

Wagner, M. (1994) *Pursuing the Birth Machine. The Search for Appropriate Technology*. ACE Graphics, Camperdown, New South Wales.

Waitzkin, H. (1979) A Marxian interpretation of the growth and development of coronary care technology. *American Journal of Public Health*, **69**, 1260–67.

Waitzkin, H. (1980) The Western social order. Letter to the Editor. *American Journal of Public Health*, **70** (4), 436–8.

Walker, P. (1990) Episiotomy: issues for practice. *Nursing*, **4** (15), 18–22.

Walker, W. P., Farine, D., Rolbin, S. H. & Ritchie, J. W. K. (1991) Epidural anesthesia, episiotomy and obstetric laceration. *Obstetrics and Gynecology*, **77** (May), 668–71.

Walters, R. (1981) Episiotomy. *Nursing Times*, (Suppl. 14) (16 September).

Webster, J. (1903) *A Text-book of Obstetrics*. W. B. Saunders and Co., Philadelphia.

Wendt, W. P. & Wolfgram, R. (1961) Episirectomy. *Obstetrics and Gynecology*, **18** (5), 626–30.

Wertz, D. (1983) What birth has done for doctors: a historical view. *Women and Health*, **8**, 7–24.

Wertz, R. & Wertz, D. (1979) *Lying-in: A History of Childbirth in America*. Schocken Books, New York.

Wertz, R. & Wertz, D. (1989) *Lying-in: A History of Childbirth in America*, expanded edn. Yale University Press, New Haven.

Whitted, G. (1981) Medical technology diffusion and its effect on the modern hospital. *Health Care Management Review*, **6** (2), 45–54.

Wilcox, L., Strobino, D., Baruffi, G. & Dellinger, W. (1989) Episiotomy and its role in the incidence of perineal lacerations in a maternity center and a tertiary hospital obstetric service. *American Journal of Obstetrics and Gynecology*, **160** (May), 1047–52.

Wilcox, R. (1885) The operation of episiotomy. *New York Medical Journal*, **42** (15 August), 176–80.

Wilkerson, V. (1984) The use of episiotomy in normal delivery. *Midwives Chronicle and Nursing Notes*, April, 106–110.

Williams, J. Whitridge (1906) *Obstetrics: A Text-book for the Use of Students and Practitioners*, 1st edn. D. Appleton and Co., New York.

Williams, J. Whitridge (1920) Discussion of DeLee's paper entitled 'The prophylactic forceps operation'. *American Journal of Obstetrics and Gynecology*, **1** (11), 77.

Williams, J. Whitridge (1926) *Obstetrics: A Text-book for the Use of Students and Practitioners*, 5th edn. D. Appleton and Co., New York.

Williams, J. Whitridge (1930) *Obstetrics: A Text-book for the Use of Students and Practitioners*, 6th edn. D. Appleton and Co., New York.

Willmott, J. (1979) No need to flaw the pelvic floor. Viewpoint. *Nursing Mirror*, 29 March, 31.

Willmott, J. (1980) Too many episiotomies. *Midwives Chronicle and Nursing Notes*, February, 46–8.

Willmott, J. (1981) Too many episiotomies. In: *Episiotomy. Physical and Emotional Aspects.* (ed. S. Kitzinger), pp. 25–9. National Childbirth Trust, London.

Wilson, J. R. (1984) Obstetric care. The effects of consumerism. Guest Editorial. *Postgraduate Medicine*, **75** (March), 15, 16, 21, 24–6.

Wilson, M. C., Hayward, R. S. A., Tunis, S. R., Bass, E. B. & Guyatt, G. (for the Evidence-Based Medicine Working Group) (1995) Users' guides to the medical literature, VIII: how to use clinical practice guidelines, B: what are the recommendations and will they help you in caring for your patients? *Journal of the American Medical Association*, **274**, 1630–32.

Woinarski, J. E. (1982) Episiotomy. Letter to the Editor. *British Medical Journal*, **284** (20 February), 595.

Woods, N. F. & Catanzaro, M. (1988) *Nursing Research*. Mosby, St Louis.

World Health Organization (1985) Appropriate technology for birth. *Lancet*, 24 August, 436–7.

Wynn, R. (1965) Concerning his method for protection of the perineum (translated from G. v. Ritgen). *American Journal of Obstetrics and Gynecology*, **93** (October), 421–33.

Yarrow, L. (1982) 20 Questions About Birth and Delivery. *Parents*, **57** (January), 62–7.

Young, D. (1982) *Changing Childbirth. Family Birth in Hospital*. Childbirth Graphics, New York.

Young, D. (ed.) (1983) *Obstetrical Intervention and Technology in the 1980s*. Haworth Press, New York.

Yunker, B. (1975) Delivery procedures that endanger a baby's life. Are doctors interfering too much with the natural process of giving birth? Many women – and some leading obstetricians – feel they are. *Good Housekeeping*, **181** (August), 56, 58, 61.

Zander, L. I. (1982) Episiotomy: has familiarity bred contempt? Editorial. *Journal of the Royal College of General Practitioners*, **32** (July), 400–401.

Zondervan, K. T., Buitendijk, S. E., Anthony, S., Van Rijssel, E. J. C. & Verkerk, P. H. (1995) Frequentie en determinanten van episiotomie in de tweedelijnsverloskunde in Nederl. *Ned Tijdschr Geneeskd*, **139** (449–52).

Index

Author Index